BMAT Practice Papers

Volume Two

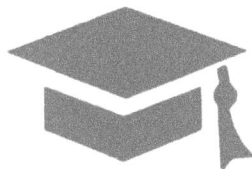

UniAdmissions

ISBN 978-1-912557-22-6

Published by *RAR Medical Services Limited*
www.uniadmissions.co.uk
info@uniadmissions.co.uk
Tel: 0208 068 0438

BMAT Practice Papers

4 Full Papers & Solutions

Matthew Williams
Rohan Agarwal

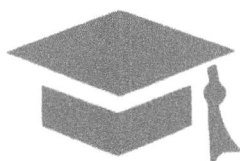

UniAdmissions

About the Authors

Matthew is **Resources Editor** at *UniAdmissions* and a final year medical student at St Catherine's College, Oxford. As the first student from Barry Comprehensive School in South Wales to receive a place on the Oxford medicine course he embraced all aspects of university life, both social and academic. Matt Scored in the **top 5% for his UKCAT and BMAT** to secure his offer at the University of Oxford.

Matthew has worked with UniAdmissions since 2014 – tutoring several applicants successfully into Oxbridge and Russell group universities. His work has been published in international scientific journals and he has presented his research at conferences across the globe. In his spare time, Matt enjoys playing rugby and golf.

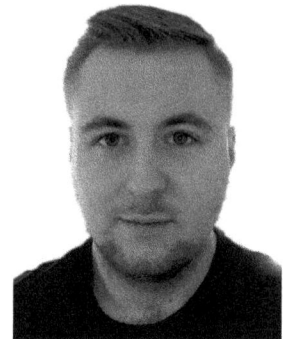

Rohan is the **Director of Operations** at *UniAdmissions* and is responsible for its technical and commercial arms. He graduated from Gonville and Caius College, Cambridge and is a fully qualified doctor. Over the last five years, he has tutored hundreds of successful Oxbridge and Medical applicants. He has also authored twenty books on admissions tests and interviews.

Rohan has taught physiology to undergraduate medical students and interviewed medical school applicants for Cambridge. He has published research on bone physiology and writes education articles for the Independent and Huffington Post. In his spare time, Rohan enjoys playing the piano and table tennis.

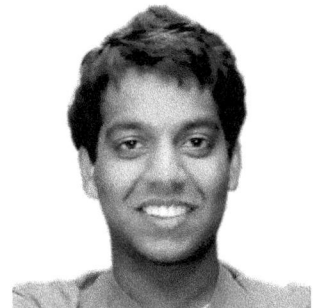

INTRODUCTION

The Basics

The BioMedical Admissions Test (BMAT) is the 2-hour written aptitude exam taken by students applying for Medicine, Biomedical Sciences, Dentistry, and Veterinary Medicine courses at the most competitive universities.

It is a highly time pressured exam that forces you to apply GCSE and A-level knowledge in ways you have never thought about before. In this respect simply remembering solutions taught in class or from past papers is not enough.

However, fear not, despite what people say, you can actually prepare for the BMAT! With a little practice you can train your brain to manipulate and apply learnt methodologies to novel problems with ease. The best way to do this is through exposure to as many past/specimen papers as you can.

Preparing for the BMAT

Before going any further, it's important that you understand the optimal way to prepare for the BMAT. Rather than jumping straight into doing mock papers, it's essential that you start by understanding the components and the theory behind the BMAT by using an BMAT textbook. Once you've finished the non-timed practice questions, you can progress to past BMAT papers. These are freely available online at www.uniadmissions.co.uk/bmat-past-papers and serve as excellent practice. You're strongly advised to use these in combination with the *BMAT Past Worked Solutions* Book so that you can improve your weaknesses. Finally, once you've exhausted past papers, move onto the mock papers in this book.

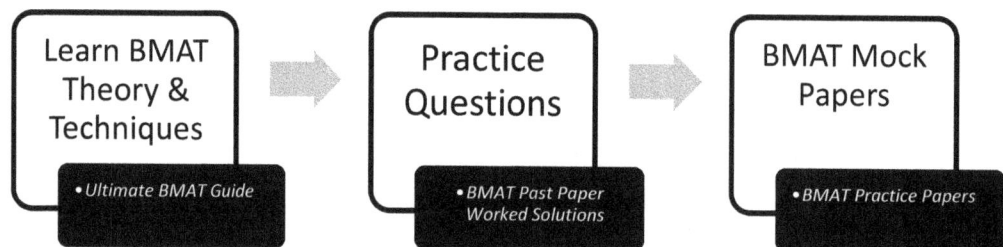

Learn BMAT Theory & Techniques	→	Practice Questions	→	BMAT Mock Papers
• *Ultimate BMAT Guide*		• *BMAT Past Paper Worked Solutions*		• *BMAT Practice Papers*

Already seen them all?

So, you've run out of past papers? Well hopefully that is where this book comes in. It contains eight unique mock papers; each compiled by expert BMAT tuors at *UniAdmissions* who scored in the top 10% nationally.

Having successfully gained a place on their course of choice, our tutors are intimately familiar with the BMAT and its associated admission procedures. So, the novel questions presented to you here are of the correct style and difficulty to continue your revision and stretch you to meet the demands of the BMAT.

General Advice

Start Early

It is much easier to prepare if you practice little and often. Start your preparation well in advance; ideally 10 weeks but at the latest within a month. This way you will have plenty of time to complete as many papers as you wish to feel comfortable and won't have to panic and cram just before the test, which is a much less effective and more stressful way to learn. In general, an early start will give you the opportunity to identify the complex issues and work at your own pace.

Prioritise

Some questions in sections can be long and complex – and given the intense time pressure you need to know your limits. It is essential that you don't get stuck with very difficult questions. If a question looks particularly long or complex, mark it for review and move on. You don't want to be caught 5 questions short at the end just because you took more than 3 minutes in answering a challenging multi-step question. If a question is taking too long, choose a sensible answer and move on. Remember that each question carries equal weighting and therefore, you should adjust your timing in accordingly. With practice and discipline, you can get very good at this and learn to maximise your efficiency.

Positive Marking

There are no penalties for incorrect answers; you will gain one for each right answer and will not get one for each wrong or unanswered one. This provides you with the luxury that you can always guess should you absolutely be not able to figure out the right answer for a question or run behind time. Since each question provides you with 4 to 6 possible answers, you have a 16-25% chance of guessing correctly. Therefore, if you aren't sure (and are running short of time), then make an educated guess and move on. Before 'guessing' you should try to eliminate a couple of answers to increase your chances of getting the question correct. For example, if a question has 5 options and you manage to eliminate 2 options- your chances of getting the question increase from 20% to 33%!

Avoid losing easy marks on other questions because of poor exam technique. Similarly, if you have failed to finish the exam, take the last 10 seconds to guess the remaining questions to at least give yourself a chance of getting them right.

Practice

This is the best way of familiarising yourself with the style of questions and the timing for this section. Although the exam will essentially only test GCSE level knowledge, you are unlikely to be familiar with the style of questions in all sections when you first encounter them. Therefore, you want to be comfortable at using this before you sit the test.

Practising questions will put you at ease and make you more comfortable with the exam. The more comfortable you are, the less you will panic on the test day and the more likely you are to score highly. Initially, work through the questions at your own pace, and spend time carefully reading the questions and looking at any additional data. When it becomes closer to the test, **make sure you practice the questions under exam conditions**.

Past Papers

Official past papers and answers from 2003 onwards are freely available online on our website at www.uniadmissions.co.uk/bmat-past-papers. Keep in mind that the specification was changed in 2009 so some things asked in earlier papers may not be representative of the content that is currently examinable in the BMAT. In general, **it is worth doing at least all the papers from 2009 onwards**. Time permitting; you can work backwards from 2009 although there is little point doing the section 3 essays pre-2009 as they are significantly different to the current style of essays.

You will undoubtedly get stuck when doing some past paper questions – they are designed to be tricky and the answer schemes don't offer any explanations. Thus, **you're highly advised to acquire a copy of** *BMAT Past Paper Worked Solutions* – a free ebook is available online (see the back of this book for more details).

Repeat Questions

When checking through answers, pay particular attention to questions you have got wrong. If there is a worked answer, look through that carefully until you feel confident that you understand the reasoning, and then repeat the question without help to check that you can do it. If only the answer is given, have another look at the question and try to work out why that answer is correct. This is the best way to learn from your mistakes, and means you are less likely to make similar mistakes when it comes to the test. The same applies for questions which you were unsure of and made an educated guess which was correct, even if you got it right. When working through this book, **make sure you highlight any questions you are unsure of**, this means you know to spend more time looking over them once marked.

No Calculators

You aren't permitted to use calculators in the exam – thus, it is essential that you have strong numerical skills. For instance, you should be able to rapidly convert between percentages, decimals and fractions. You will seldom get questions that would require calculators, but you would be expected to be able to arrive at a sensible estimate. Consider for example:

Estimate 3.962 x 2.322;

3.962 is approximately 4 and 2.323 is approximately 2.33 = 7/3.

Thus, $3.962 \times 2.322 \approx 4 \times \frac{7}{3} = \frac{28}{3} = 9.33$

Since you will rarely be asked to perform difficult calculations, you can use this as a signpost of if you are tackling a question correctly. For example, when solving a physics question, you end up having to divide 8,079 by 357- this should raise alarm bells as calculations in the BMAT are rarely this difficult.

A word on timing...

"If you had all day to do your exam, you would get 100%. But you don't."
Whilst this isn't completely true, it illustrates a very important point. Once you've practiced and know how to answer the questions, the clock is your biggest enemy. This seemingly obvious statement has one very important consequence. **The way to improve your score is to improve your speed.** There is no magic bullet. But there are a great number of techniques that, with practice, will give you significant time gains, allowing you to answer more questions and score more marks.

Timing is tight throughout – **mastering timing is the first key to success**. Some candidates choose to work as quickly as possible to save up time at the end to check back, but this is generally not the best way to do it. Often questions can have a lot of information in them – each time you start answering a question it takes time to get familiar with the instructions and information. By splitting the question into two sessions (the first run-through and the return-to-check) you double the amount of time you spend on familiarising yourself with the data, as you have to do it twice instead of only once. This costs valuable time. In addition, candidates who do check back may spend 2–3 minutes doing so and yet not make any actual changes. Whilst this can be reassuring, it is a false reassurance as it is unlikely to have a significant effect on your actual score. Therefore, it is usually best to pace yourself very steadily, aiming to spend the same amount of time on each question and finish the final question in a section just as time runs out. This reduces the time spent on re-familiarising with questions and maximises the time spent on the first attempt, gaining more marks.

It is essential that you don't get stuck with the hardest questions – no doubt there will be some. In the time spent answering only one of these you may miss out on answering three easier questions. If a question is taking too long, choose a sensible answer and move on. Never see this as giving up or in any way failing, rather it is the smart way to approach a test with a tight time limit. With practice and discipline, you can get very good at this and learn to maximise your efficiency. It is not about being a hero and aiming for full marks – this is almost impossible and very much unnecessary (even Oxbridge will regard any score higher than 7 as exceptional). It is about maximising your efficiency and gaining the maximum possible number of marks within the time you have.

Use the Options:

Some questions may try to overload you with information. When presented with large tables and data, it's essential you look at the answer options so you can focus your mind. This can allow you to reach the correct answer a lot more quickly. Consider the example below:

The table below shows the results of a study investigating antibiotic resistance in staphylococcus populations. A single staphylococcus bacterium is chosen at random from a similar population. Resistance to any one antibiotic is independent of resistance to others.

Calculate the probability that the bacterium selected will be resistant to all four drugs.

A 1 in 10^6
B 1 in 10^{12}
C 1 in 10^{20}
D 1 in 10^{25}
E 1 in 10^{30}
F 1 in 10^{35}

Antibiotic	Number of Bacteria tested	Number of Resistant Bacteria
Benzyl-penicillin	10^{11}	98
Chloramphenicol	10^9	1200
Metronidazole	10^8	256
Erythromycin	10^5	2

Looking at the options first makes it obvious that there is **no need to calculate exact values**- only in powers of 10. This makes your life a lot easier. If you hadn't noticed this, you might have spent well over 90 seconds trying to calculate the exact value when it wasn't even being asked for.

In other cases, you may actually be able to use the options to arrive at the solution quicker than if you had tried to solve the question as you normally would. Consider the example below:

A region is defined by the two inequalities: $x - y^2 > 1$ and $xy > 1$. Which of the following points is in the defined region?

A. (10,3)
B. (10,2)
C. (-10,3)
D. (-10,2)
E. (-10,-3)

Whilst it's possible to solve this question both algebraically or graphically by manipulating the identities, by far **the quickest way is to actually use the options**. Note that options C, D and E violate the second inequality, narrowing down to answer to either A or B. For A: $10 - 3^2 = 1$ and thus this point is on the boundary of the defined region and not actually in the region. Thus the answer is B (as 10-4 = 6 > 1.)

In general, it pays dividends to look at the options briefly and see if they can be help you arrive at the question more quickly. Get into this habit early – it may feel unnatural at first but it's guaranteed to save you time in the long run.

Keywords

If you're stuck on a question; pay particular attention to the options that contain key modifiers like "**always**", "**only**", "**all**" as examiners like using them to test if there are any gaps in your knowledge. E.g. the statement "arteries carry oxygenated blood" would normally be true; "All arteries carry oxygenated blood" would be false because the pulmonary artery carries deoxygenated blood.

Manage your Time:

It is highly likely that you will be juggling your revision alongside your normal school studies. Whilst it is tempting to put your A-levels on the back burner falling behind in your school subjects is not a good idea, don't forget that to meet the conditions of your offer should you get one you will need at least one A*. So, time management is key!

Make sure you set aside a dedicated 90 minutes (and much more closer to the exam) to commit to your revision each day. The key here is not to sacrifice too many of your extracurricular activities, everybody needs some down time, but instead to be efficient. Take a look at our list of top tips for increasing revision efficiency below:

1. Create a comfortable work station
2. Declutter and stay tidy
3. Treat yourself to some nice stationery
4. See if music works for you → if not, find somewhere peaceful and quiet to work
5. Turn off your mobile or at least put it into silent mode
6. Silence social media alerts
7. Keep the TV off and out of sight
8. Stay organised with to do lists and revision timetables – more importantly, stick to them!
9. Keep to your set study times and don't bite off more than you can chew
10. Study while you're commuting
11. Adopt a positive mental attitude
12. Get into a routine
13. Consider forming a study group to focus on the harder exam concepts
14. Plan rest and reward days into your timetable – these are excellent incentive for you to stay on track with your study plans!

Keep Fit & Eat Well:

'A car won't work if you fill it with the wrong fuel' - your body is exactly the same. You cannot hope to perform unless you remain fit and well. The best way to do this is not underestimate the importance of healthy eating. Beige, starchy foods will make you sluggish; instead start the day with a hearty breakfast like porridge. Aim for the recommended 'five a day' intake of fruit/veg and stock up on the oily fish or blueberries – the so called "super foods".

When hitting the books, it's essential to keep your brain hydrated. If you get dehydrated you'll find yourself lethargic and possibly developing a headache, neither of which will do any favours for your revision. Invest in a good water bottle that you know the total volume of and keep sipping through the day. Don't forget that the amount of water you should be aiming to drink varies depending on your mass, so calculate your own personal recommended intake as follows: 30 ml per kg per day.

It is well known that exercise boosts your wellbeing and instils a sense of discipline. All of which will reflect well in your revision. It's well worth devoting half an hour a day to some exercise, get your heart rate up, break a sweat, and get those endorphins flowing.

Sleep

It's no secret that when revising you need to keep well rested. Don't be tempted to stay up late revising as sleep actually plays an important part in consolidating long term memory. Instead aim for a minimum of 7 hours good sleep each night, in a dark room without any glow from electronic appliances. Install flux (https://justgetflux.com) on your laptop to prevent your computer from disrupting your circadian rhythm. Aim to go to bed the same time each night and no hitting snooze on the alarm clock in the morning!

Revision Timetable

Still struggling to get organised? Then try filling in the example revision timetable below, remember to factor in enough time for short breaks, and stick to it! Remember to schedule in several breaks throughout the day and actually use them to do something you enjoy e.g. TV, reading, YouTube etc.

	8AM	0AM	2PM	4PM	6PM	3PM
MONDAY						
TUESDAY						
'HURSDAY						
FRIDAY						
ATURDAY						
SUNDAY						
EXAMPLE DAY	School		Biology	Critical	vsics	

ɒ tip! Ensure that you take a watch that can show you the time in seconds into the exam. This will allow have a much more accurate idea of the time you're spending on a question. In general, if you've spent 0 seconds on a section 1 question or >90 seconds on a section 2 questions – move on regardless of how close you think you are to solving it.

Getting the most out of Mock Papers

Mock exams can prove invaluable if tackled correctly. Not only do they encourage you to start revision earlier, they also allow you to **practice and perfect your revision technique**. They are often the best way of improving your knowledge base or reinforcing what you have learnt. Probably the best reason for attempting mock papers is to familiarise yourself with the exam conditions of the BMAT as they are particularly tough.

Start Revision Earlier

Thirty five percent of students agree that they procrastinate to a degree that is detrimental to their exam performance. This is partly explained by the fact that they often seem a long way in the future. In the scientific literature this is well recognised, Dr. Piers Steel, an expert on the field of motivation states that *'the further away an event is, the less impact it has on your decisions'*.

Mock exams are therefore a way of giving you a target to work towards and motivate you in the run up to the real thing – every time you do one treat it as the real deal! If you do well then it's a reassuring sign; if you do poorly then it will motivate you to work harder (and earlier!).

Practice and perfect revision techniques

In case you haven't realised already, revision is a skill all to itself, and can take some time to learn. For example, the most common revision techniques including **highlighting and/or re-reading are quite ineffective** ways of committing things to memory. Unless you are thinking critically about something you are much less likely to remember it or indeed understand it.

Mock exams, therefore allow you to test your revision strategies as you go along. Try spacing out your revision sessions so you have time to forget what you have learnt in-between. This may sound counterintuitive but the second time you remember it for longer. Try teaching another student what you have learnt, this forces you to structure the information in a logical way that may aid memory. Always try to question what you have learnt and appraise its validity. Not only does this aid memory but it is also a useful skill for BMAT section 3, Oxbridge interview, and beyond.

Improve your knowledge

The act of applying what you have learnt reinforces that piece of knowledge. A question may ask you to think about a relatively basic concept in a novel way (not cited in textbooks), and so deepen your understanding. Exams rarely test word for word what is in the syllabus, so when running through mock papers try to understand how the basic facts are applied and tested in the exam. As you go through the mocks or past papers take note of your performance and see if you consistently under-perform in specific areas, thus highlighting areas for future study.

Get familiar with exam conditions

Pressure can cause all sorts of trouble for even the most brilliant students. The BMAT is a particularly time pressured exam with high stakes – your future (without exaggerating) does depend on your result to a great extent. The real key to the BMAT is overcoming this pressure and remaining calm to allow you to think efficiently.

Mock exams are therefore an excellent opportunity to devise and perfect your own exam techniques to beat the pressure and meet the demands of the exam. **Don't treat mock exams like practice questions – it's imperative you do them under time conditions.**

Remember! It's better that you make all the mistakes you possibly can now in mock papers and then learn from them so as not to repeat them in the real exam.

Things to have done before using this book

Do the ground work

➢ Read in detail: the background, methods, and aims of the BMAT as well logistical considerations such as how to take the BMAT in practice. A good place to start is a BMAT textbook like *The Ultimate BMAT Guide* (flick to the back to get a free copy!) which covers all the groundwork but it's also worth looking through the official BMAT site (www.admissionstesting.org/bmat).

➢ It is generally a good idea to start re-capping all your GCSE maths and science.

➢ Practice substituting formulas together to reach a more useful one expressing known variables e.g. $P = IV$ and $V = IR$ can be combined to give $P = V^2/R$ and $P = I^2R$. Remember that calculators are not permitted in the exam, so get comfortable doing more complex long addition, multiplication, division, and subtraction.

➢ Get comfortable rapidly converting between percentages, decimals, and fractions.

➢ Practice developing logical arguments and structuring essays with an obvious introduction, main body, and ending.

➢ These are all things which are easiest to do alongside your revision for exams before the summer break. Not only gaining a head start on your BMAT revision but also complimenting your year 12 studies well.

➢ Discuss scientific problems with others - propose experiments and state what you think the result would be. Be ready to defend your argument. This will rapidly build your scientific understanding for section 2 but also prepare you well for an oxbridge interview.

➢ Read through the BMAT syllabus before you start tackling whole papers. This is absolutely essential. It contains several stated formulae, constants, and facts that you are expected to apply - or may just be an answer in their own right. Familiarising yourself with the syllabus is also a quick way of teaching yourself the additional information other exam boards may learn which you do not. Sifting through the whole BMAT syllabus is a time-consuming process so we have done it for you. **Be sure to flick through the syllabus checklist** later on, which also doubles up as a great revision aid for the night before!

Ease in gently

With the ground work laid, there's still no point in adopting exam conditions straight away. Instead invest in a beginner's guide to the BMAT, which will not only describe in detail the background and theory of the exam, but take you through section by section what is expected. *The Ultimate BMAT Guide: 800 Practice Questions* is the most popular BMAT textbook – you can get a free copy by flicking to the back of this book.

When you are ready to move on to past papers, take your time and puzzle your way through all the questions. Really try to understand solutions. A past paper question won't be repeated in your real exam, so don't rote learn methods or facts. Instead, focus on applying prior knowledge to formulate your own approach.

If you're really struggling and have to take a sneak peek at the answers, then practice thinking of alternative solutions, or arguments for essays. It is unlikely that your answer will be more elegant or succinct than the model answer, but it is still a good task for encouraging creativity with your thinking. Get used to thinking outside the box!

Accelerate and Intensify

Start adopting exam conditions after you've done two past papers. Don't forget that **it's the time pressure that makes the BMAT hard** – if you had as long as you wanted to sit the exam you would probably get 100%. If you're struggling to find comprehensive answers to past papers then *BMAT Past Papers Worked Solutions* contains detailed explained answers to every BMAT past paper question and essay (flick to the back to get a free copy).

Doing all the past papers from 2009 – present is a good target for your revision. Note that the BMAT syllabus changed in 2009 so questions before this date may no longer be relevant. In any case, choose a paper and proceed with strict exam conditions. Take a short break and then mark your answers before reviewing your progress. For revision purposes, as you go along, keep track of those questions that you guess – these are equally as important to review as those you get wrong.

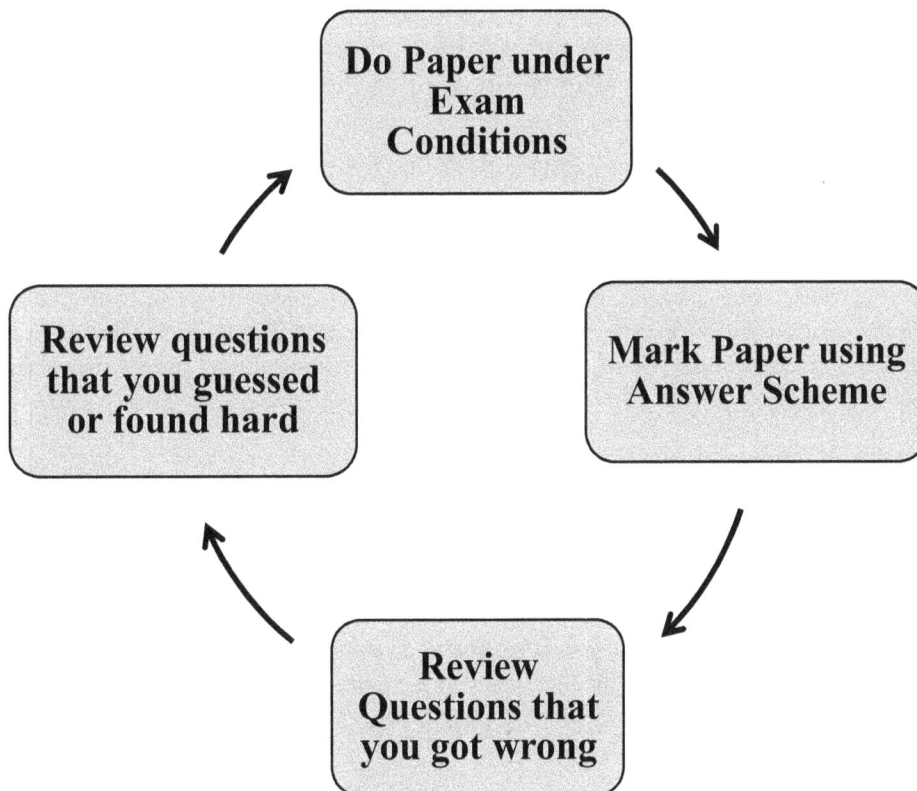

```
        ┌─────────────────────┐
        │   Do Paper under    │
        │        Exam         │
        │     Conditions      │
        └─────────────────────┘

┌──────────────────────┐      ┌──────────────────────┐
│  Review questions    │      │   Mark Paper using   │
│  that you guessed     │      │    Answer Scheme     │
│   or found hard       │      │                      │
└──────────────────────┘      └──────────────────────┘

        ┌─────────────────────┐
        │       Review        │
        │   Questions that    │
        │    you got wrong    │
        └─────────────────────┘
```

Once you've exhausted all the past papers, move on to tackling the unique mock papers in this book. In general, you should aim to complete one to two mock papers every night in the ten days preceding your exam.

Section 1: An Overview

What will you be tested on?	No. of Questions	Duration
Generic skills in problem solving, understanding arguments, and critical thinking.	32 MCQs	60 Minutes

This is the first section of the BMAT, comprising what most people describe as the classic IQ test style questions. Giving you one hour to answer 35 questions testing your ability to think critically, solve problems, and handle data. Breaking things down you realise that you are left with approximately 110 seconds per question. Remember though that this not only includes reasoning your answers, but also reading passages of text and/or analysing diagrams or graphs.

Not all the questions are of equal difficulty and so as you work through the past material it is certainly worth learning to recognise quickly which questions you need to skip to avoid getting bogged down. If it comes to it and you do not have enough time to go back to any skipped questions at the end, you always have a 20% chance of getting the answer correct with a guess!

Critical thinking questions

These types of question will generally present you with a passage of text or a methodology for an experiment and ask you to do one of three things: identify a conclusion, identify and assumption or flaw, or give an argument to either strengthen or weaken the statement.

The ability to filter through irrelevant material is essential with these questions as well as a solid grasp of the English language. Remember to only use the information given to you in your reasoning and never be too general with your conclusions – seek direct evidence in the information given. Critical thinking questions are definitely an example of when it is **best to read the question first**!

Problem solving questions

The problems in section 1 are often very wordy and complex, therefore it is often useful to turn the prose of the question into a series of equations. For example, being able to turn the sentence "Megan is half as tall as Elin" into "2M = E" should become second nature to you. Trial and error is not a method you should adopt for any questions in section 1 as it is far too time consuming.

As you are working through the preparation material try to get used to recognising which questions can be aided by drawing a quick diagram. This could apply to questions asking about timetables, orders, sequences, or spatial relationships. Remember it doesn't have to be pretty, merely help you organise your thoughts!

Section 2: An Overview

What will you be tested on?	No. of Questions	Duration
The ability to apply scientific knowledge typically covered in school Science and Mathematics by 16	27 MCQs	30 Minutes

If you're short of time, then section 2 is where to focus. Undoubtedly the most time pressured section of the BMAT (requiring you to answer a question a minute) but also the section where candidates improve the fastest. Section 2 draws on your GCSE knowledge of biology, chemistry, physics, and maths.

It is important to remember that this is **GCSE knowledge taken from ALL exam boards**. So, you may find information that you are not familiar with if it was ignored by your exam board. To make sure you have a comprehensive knowledge of all the required material be sure to run through the section 2 revision checklists on the next few pages.

Biology

Generally, the biology questions require the least amount of time and are often where you can rely on making up lost time from harder questions. Most of biology questions rely on you being able to recall facts rather than interpret data or solve equations, so some good old-fashioned text book revision will prepare you well for these questions.

Chemistry

If you're taking the BMAT you will undoubtedly be studying chemistry at A-level as it is a requirement of all medical schools. Conceptually therefore, you should be in the clear, however, balancing complex equations or processing lengthy calculations can be time consuming.

Practicing with mock papers is essentially in combating this – really focus on extracting what the question is asking for as quickly as possible. In addition to the equations on the subsequent pages you must be comfortable with converting between litres, dm^3, cm^3, and mm^3 as well as using Avogadro's constant in calculations.

Physics

Physics is by far the most common subject that students drop moving on to AS-level, meaning these questions are the most poorly answered. There is a large variation in physics specifications between GCSE exam boards, so **before you do anything else read through the BMAT syllabus and commit all the stated equations and constants to memory** (helpfully highlighted in bold type on the revision checklist).

Physics questions will almost always require a two-step solution, normally forcing you to combine and re-arrange equations. All answers must be given in SI units which actually benefits you, by looking at the units you can often derive the equation – for example speed in m/s is calculated as distance(m) / time(s). It is also worth becoming fluent with the terminology for orders of magnitude in measurements (see right).

Factor	Text	Symbol
10^{12}	Tera	T
10^9	Giga	G
10^6	Mega	M
10^3	Kilo	k
10^2	Hecto	h
10^{-1}	Deci	d
10^{-2}	Centi	c
10^{-3}	Milli	m
10^{-6}	Micro	μ
10^{-9}	Nano	n
10^{-12}	Pico	p

Maths

Maths is the single most important component of section 2, a question topic in its own right but also applied in chemistry, physics, and section 1. Just remember to limit yourself to GCSE knowledge in the maths questions and don't overcomplicate things. As a bare minimum for preparation you should practice applying the quadratic formula, completing the square, and finding the difference between 2 squares.

Section 2: Revision Checklist

MATHS

Syllabus Point	What to Know
1. **Units**	Standard units of mass, length, time, money, and other measures Define compound units Change freely between related standard and compound units
2. **Number**	Order positive and negative integers, decimals, and fractions Understand and use $=, \neq, \leq, \geq, <, >$ Understand and use BIDMAS Define; factor, multiple, common factor, highest common factor, least common multiple, prime number, prime factor decomposition, square, positive and negative square root, cube and cube root Use index laws to simplify multiplication and division of powers Interpret, order and calculate with numbers written in standard index form Convert between fractions, decimals and percentages Understand and use direct and indirect proportion Apply the unitary method Use surds and π in exact calculations, simplify expressions that contain surds. Calculate upper and lower bounds to contextual problems Rounding to a given number of decimal places or significant figures
3. **Ratio and Proportion**	Use scale factors, diagrams, and maps Express a quantity as a fracation of another Express division of a quantity in two parts as a ratio Understand and use proportion Define percentage Work with percentages greater than 100% Solve problems using percentage change Appreciate why percentage can be used rather than a raw number
4. **Algebra**	Simplify rational expressions by cancelling or factorising and cancelling Set up quadratic equations and solve them by factorising Know the quadratic formula Set up and use equations to solve problems involving direct and indirect proportion Use linear expressions to describe the nth term of a sequence Use Cartesian coordinates in all four quadrants Equation of a straight line, $y=mx+c$, parallel lines have the same gradient Identify pairs of parallel and perpendicular lines Graphically solve simultaneous equations Recognise and interpret graphs of simple cubic functions, the reciprocal function, trigonometric functions and the exponential function $y=kx$ for integer values of x and simple positive values of k Draw transformations of $y = f(x)$ [$(y=af(x), y=f(ax), y=f(x)+a, y=f(x-a)$ only] Deduce expressions to calculate the nth term in a sequence
5. **Geometry**	Recall and use properties of angle at a point, on a straight line, perpendicular lines and opposite angles at a vertex, and the sums of the interior and exterior angles of polygons Understand congruence and similarity Use Pythagoras' theorem in 2-D and 3-D Use the trigonometric ratios, between 0° and 180°, to solve problems in 2-D and 3-D Understand and construct geometrical proofs, including using circle theorems: **a. the angle subtended at the circumference in a semicircle is a right angle** **b. the tangent at any point on a circle is perpendicular to the radius at that point** Describe and transform 2-D shapes using single or combined rotations, reflections, translations, or enlargements, including the use of vector notation

6.	**Measures**	Use conventional terms and notation Calculate perimeters and areas of shapes made from triangles, rectangles, and other shapes, find circumferences and areas of circles, including arcs and sectors Apply the standard circle theorems concerning angles, radii, tangents, and chords: • Angle subtended at the centre is twice the angle subtended at the circumference • Angle in a semicircle is 90° • Angles in the same segment are equal • Angle between a tangent and a chord (alternate segment theorem) • Angle between a radius and a tangent is 90° • Properties of cyclic quadrilaterals Calculate the volumes and surface areas of prisms, pyramids, spheres, cylinders, cones and solids made from cubes and cuboids (formulae given for the sphere and cone) Use vectors, including the sum of two vectors, algebraically and graphically Discuss the inaccuracies of measurements Understand and use three-figure bearings
7.	**Statistics**	Identify possible sources of bias in experimental methodology Discrete vs. continuous data Interpret cumulative frequency tables and graphs, box plots and histograms Define mean, median, mode, modal class, range, and inter-quartile range Interpret scatter diagrams and recognise correlation, drawing and using lines of best fit Compare sets of data by using statistical measures
8.	**Probability**	List all the outcomes for single and combined events Identify different mutually exclusive outcomes and know that the sum of the probabilities of all these outcomes is 1 Construct and use Venn diagrams Know when to add or multiply two probabilities, and understand conditional probability Understand the use of tree diagrams to represent outcomes of combined events Compare experimental and theoretical probabilities Understand that if an experiment is repeated, the outcome may be different

BIOLOGY

Syllabus Point	What to Know
1. **Cells**	Differences in cellular structure and function between: -Animals: cell membrane, cytoplasm, nucleus, mitochondrion -Plants: cell membrane, cytoplasm, nucleus, cell wall, chloroplast, mitochondrion, vacuole -Bacteria: cell membrane, cytoplasm, cell wall, no true nucleus Multiple cells form tissues, several tissues form an organ
2. **Movement Across Membranes**	Difference between diffusion, osmosis, and active transport Role of cellular proteins Need for mitochondria in active transport
3. **Cell Division & Sex**	Define mitosis vs. meiosis Asexual vs. sexual reproduction Sex determination: females XX, males XY Calculate gender ratio
4. **Inheritance**	Role of nucleus in cell function Define genes, alleles, dominant, recessive, heterozygous, homozygous, phenotype, and genotype Use monohybrid crosses and family trees to calculate ratios/percentages Cystic fibrosis, polydactyly, and Huntington's
5. **DNA**	Chromosomes Structure of DNA Protein synthesis from DNA base triplets
6. **Gene Technologies**	Methods of experimental gene insertion Roles of stem cells: embryonic vs. adult
7. **Variation**	Natural selection: variation, differential survival based on adaptation, only those best adapted survive to reproduce Antibiotic resistance (MRSA) Genetic vs. environmental causes of variation Extinction occurs when organisms can't adapt quickly enough
8. **Enzymes**	Define biological catalyst Mechanism of action: lock and key vs. induced fit Effects of temperature and pH The role of amylase, protease, and lipase
9. **Animal Physiology**	Define and describe aerobic and anaerobic respiration Define homeostasis Negative vs. positive feedback Regulation of blood glucose, water, and temperature Function of white blood cells Hormones: travel in blood to target organs Structure (anatomy), organisation, and function of the: -Nervous system: sensory vs. motor vs. relay neurons, reflex arcs, synapses -Respiratory system: thorax, process of ventilation and gas exchange -Circulatory system: sinoatrial node, atrioventricular node, heart rate and ECGs, differences between arteries, veins, and capillaries, blood groups -Digestive system: digestive enzymes, pH -Kidney: the nephron, role in homeostasis
10. **Ecosystems**	Food chains, energy flow Pyramids of biomass Define niche Factors affecting population growth Carbon cycle: photosynthesis, respiration, combustion, decomposition Nitrogen cycle: bacteria, nitrification, decomposition, nitrogen fixation, denitrification

CHEMISTRY

	Syllabus Point	What to Know
1.	**Atomic Structure**	Structure of the atom Relative masses and charges of protons, neutrons, and electrons Atomic vs. mass number, electron configurations Isotope definition Define A_r, calculate M_r Mass spectrometry
2.	**Periodic Table**	Organisation of periods vs. groups and metals vs. non-metals Displacement reactions and reactivity, extraction of metals from their ores Position of the alkali metals, halogens, noble gases, and transition metals, relate position to electron configuration Reactivity increases down a metal group but decreases down a non-metal group Properties of transition metals Calculate A_r from isotopic mass and abundance.
3.	**Reactions & Equations**	Conservation of matter Endothermic vs. exothermic Charges of common polyatomic cations (e.g. CO_3^{2-}) Formulate equations describing redox reactions Factors that affect the position of equilibrium in reversible reactions
4.	**Calculations**	Define the mole, convert grams to moles, **1 mole of gas = 24dm³** Percentage composition by mass of a compound, empirical vs. molecular formulae Calculate reactants in excess Calculate molar concentration **moles = (volume cm³/1000) x concentration mol dm⁻³** Titration calculation, define saturated **Percentage yield = (actual yield/predicted yield) x 100**
5.	**Redox**	Describe oxidation vs. reduction Recognise disproportionation Transfer of electrons, determine oxidation states
6.	**Bonding**	Define elements vs. compounds Ionic vs. covalent vs. metallic bonding, simple and giant covalent structures
7.	**Groups**	Alkali metals: group 1, electron donors, low melting/boiling points, store in oil, describe reaction with water, oxygen, and halogens Halogens: most reactive non-metals, establishing reactivity series with displacement reactions, reactions with silver nitrate Noble gases: least reactive elements Transition metals: position in the periodic table, properties and uses
8.	**Separation techniques**	Compounds vs. mixtures Miscible liquid separation: fractional distillation, chromatography Immiscible liquid separation: separating funnel Dissolving, filtering, distillation, and crystallisation
9.	**Acids and Bases**	Definitions and properties of strong and weak acids and bases
10.	**Rates of Reaction**	Effects of concentration, temperature, particle size, catalyst presence, and pressure Calculate loss of reactant over time, predict measurable variables from chemical equation Collision theory and activation energy Function of catalysts
11.	**Energetics**	Exothermic vs. endothermic
12.	**Electrolysis**	Define electrode, cathode, anode, and electrolyte Why DC not AC? Electrolysis of brine and electroplating using copper sulfate
13.	**Organic**	Alkanes vs. alkenes (general formulae, IUPAC terminology, saturated vs. unsaturated, combustion) Polymers: method of alkene polymerisation, define monomer, identify biodegradable and non-biodegradable polymers General formulae, chemical properties, and uses of alcohols and carboxylic acids

14. Metals	Reactivity series and displacement reactions Uses of common metals linked to their properties Extraction of metals from their ores Properties of transition metals including oxidation states, colour, and use as catalysts
15. Particle Theory	Describe the packing and movement of particles in all three states of matter Appreciate the changes in these models during a change of state (freezing, melting, evaporation, and condensation) Understand that the energy required is related to the bonding and structure
16. Chemical Tests	Know the benchside tests for: <ul><li>**Hydrogen – squeaky pop**</li><li>**Oxygen – relight a glowing splint**</li><li>**Carbon dioxide – limewater turns cloudy**</li><li>**Chlorine – litmus paper turns red then white**</li><li>**Carbonates – dilute acid**</li><li>**Halides – silver nitrate and nitric acid**</li><li>**Sulfates – barium chloride and hydrochloric acid**</li></ul>Know the positive sign for metal cations in aqueous sodium hydroxide <ul><li>Al^{3+}, Ca^{2+}, and Mg^{2+} **form a white precipitate**</li><li>Cu^{2+} **forms a blue precipitate**</li><li>Fe^{2+} **forms a green precipitate**</li><li>Fe^{3+} **forms a brown precipitate**</li></ul>Know the flame tests for cations <ul><li>**Li – crimson red**</li><li>**Na – yellow-orange**</li><li>**K – lilac**</li><li>**Ca – red-orange**</li><li>**Cu – green**</li></ul>Test for water with anhydrous copper (II) sulfate (**white to blue**)
17. Air and Water	Fractional distillation can be used to separate the components of air Know the origins and effects of greenhouse gases Know the origins and effects of gaseous pollutants Know the purpose of chlorine and fluoride ions in water treatment

PHYSICS

Syllabus Point	What to Know
1. **Electricity**	Electrostatics: charging of insulators by friction, gain of electrons induces negative charge, uses in paint spraying and dust extraction Conductors vs. insulators **Current = charge/ time** **Resistance = voltage/ current**, how to connect ammeters and voltmeters V–I graphs for a fixed resistor and a filament lamp Series vs. parallel circuits Resistors in series (but not parallel) **Voltage = energy/ charge** Basic circuit symbols and diagrams **Power = current x voltage** **Energy = power x time**
2. **Magnetism**	Properties of magnets Magnetic field due to an electric current The motor effect: $F = BIL$ Construction and operation of a DC motor Electromagnetic induction and the applications $\left(\frac{V_p}{V_s} = \frac{n_p}{n_s}\right)$ thus when 100% efficient $V_pI_p = V_sI_s$ Method of electromagnetic induction, applied to a generator
3. **Mechanics**	**Speed = distance/time**, difference between speed and velocity **Acceleration = change in velocity/time** Distance-time vs. velocity-time graphs (including calculation and interpretation of gradients and average speed) Equation of motion: $v^2 - u^2 = 2as$ Types of force Newtons laws: -First: **momentum = mass x velocity**, conservation of momentum -Second: **force = mass x acceleration, force = rate of change of momentum**, resultant force, $W = mg$, gravitational field strength (~10N/kg on Earth), free fall acceleration, terminal velocity -Third = every action has an equal and opposite reaction Elastic vs inelastic extensions Hooke's law: $F = kx$ Energy in a stretched sping: $E = \frac{1}{2}Fx = \frac{1}{2}kx^2$ **Work = force x distance** = transfer of energy **Potential energy = mgh** **Kinetic energy** $= \frac{1}{2}mv^2$ Crumple zones and road safety **Power = energy transfer/time** Conservation of energy, forms of energy, useful and wasted energy, % efficiency
4. **Thermal physics**	Conduction: factors affecting rate of conduction Convection: temperature and density of fluids Radiation: infrared, absorption and re-emission Experimental methods of determining densities
5. **Matter**	Particle models of solids, liquids, gases, and state changes Behaviour of ideal gases: **PV = constant** Understand the terms melting point, boiling point, latent heat of fusion, latent heat of vaporisation **Density = mass/volume** Compare densities of solids, liquids, and gases **Pressure = force/area** **Hydrostatic pressure = hpg**

6.	**Waves**	Transfer of energy without net movement of matter, transverse (electromagnetic) vs. longitudinal (sound) Define amplitude, wavelength, frequency ($1Hz = 1$ wave/second), and period **Frequency = 1/period** **Wave speed = frequency x wavelength** Reflection and refraction (including ray diagrams), and Doppler effect Angle in incidence = angle of reflection Production and properties of sound waves Range of human hearing is **20Hz to 20kHz** Application of ultrasound Properties of electromagnetic waves (speed of light, transverse) Distinguished by wavelength, longest to shortest: radio, microwaves, infrared, visible light, ultraviolet, x-ray, gamma Applications and dangers
7.	**Radioactivity**	Atomic structure, charges and mass of subatomic particles, ionisation Radioactive decay: alpha vs. beta vs. gamma emission, decay equations, define activity of a sample Ionising radiation: penetrating ability, ionising ability, presence of background radiation (including origin), applications and dangers Define half-life and interpret from graphs Apply half-life calculations Nuclear fission: absorption of thermal neutrons, uranium-235 (decay equation), chain reaction Nuclear fusion: hydrogen to form helium, requires significant temperature and pressure, significance as a possible energy sauce

Section 3: An Overview

What will you be tested on?	No of Questions	Duration
The ability to select, develop and organise ideas, and to communicate them in writing, concisely and effectively.	One writing task from a choice of three questions	30 minutes

Section 3 asks you to write one A4 page essay from a choice of 3 essay questions. Obviously certain questions require some background understanding to be able to interpret the question, but essentially the only skill being tested is your ability to construct a logical and coherent argument (whether it's right or wrong does not matter).

So, the aim is not to squeeze as much as you can onto the page but rather present your opinions supported with evidence, and then tie everything together with a logical conclusion answering the initial question. Be warned that irrelevant material for the sake of filling space may actually negatively affect your score! You're scored 0 – 5 for the content of your essay and A – E for the quality of your written communication.

The theory behind the essay

Most BMAT section 3 questions all follow the same syntax. Firstly, they present a quote or statement, then ask you: 1) explain it, 2) argue for or against it, and finally 3) "to what extent" do you agree.

1) is the easy bit and shouldn't exceed three lines of text, this is your chance to lay the grounding for your essay – if you are unsure of what a word means, or the statement is ambiguous, categorically define it here and say this is what all your arguments are based around.

2) should comprise the main body of your essay. Here you need to demonstrate your understanding of the concept by offering critical insight strengthened by any evidence you are aware of. You should aim to explore two distinct ideas and acknowledge their counter arguments.

3) is really the chance for your personality to shine through. Don't be vague or unimaginative! Be brave and make a bold statement that can be derived from considering all the points you have discussed, reasoning both sides of the argument.

Structuring the essay

With such tight time constraints there is no time to devise a complex essay weaving your points through the paragraphs – and for examiners reading 100 essays a night it's just confusing. Keep it simple and follow the age old classic model described below:

Introduction: *say what you're going to say and how you're going to say it*. This is your opportunity to explain the quote/statement, give any relevant background information needed to validate your arguments, and finally indicate the logical flow of your arguments to follow.

Main body of text: *say it*. Now is the time to develop your points and insert your own personal opinions (validated by fact!) with examples if you have them. A good system to follow for each point you make is point → evidence → evaluate. Don't forget to link your paragraphs and compare arguments to show a deeper level of understanding.

Conclusion: *say what you've said*. Here you draw everything to a close. You should not introduce any new information but rather summarise your main points to leave your final take home message. Don't forget to answer the question explicitly at the end. Often a nice way to end is by asking a relevant question back to the reader that your argument brings to light.

How to use this Book

If you have done everything this book has described so far then you should be well equipped to meet the demands of the BMAT, and therefore **the mock papers in the rest of this book should ONLY be completed under exam conditions**.

This means:

➢ Absolute silence – no TV or music
➢ Absolute focus – no distractions such as eating your dinner
➢ Strict time constraints – no pausing half way through
➢ No checking the answers as you go
➢ Give yourself a maximum of three minutes between sections – keep the pressure up
➢ Complete the entire paper before marking
➢ Mark harshly

In practice this means setting aside two hours in an evening to find a quiet spot without interruptions and tackle the paper. Completing one mock paper every evening in the week running up to the exam would be an ideal target.

➢ Tackle the paper as you would in the exam.
➢ Return to mark your answers, but mark harshly if there's any ambiguity.
➢ Highlight any areas of concern.
➢ If warranted read up on the areas you felt you underperformed to reinforce your knowledge.
➢ If you inadvertently learnt anything new by muddling through a question, go and tell somebody about it to reinforce what you've discovered.

Finally relax… the BMAT is an exhausting exam, concentrating so hard continually for two hours will take its toll. So, being able to relax and switch off is essential to keep yourself sharp for exam day! Make sure you reward yourself after you finish marking your exam.

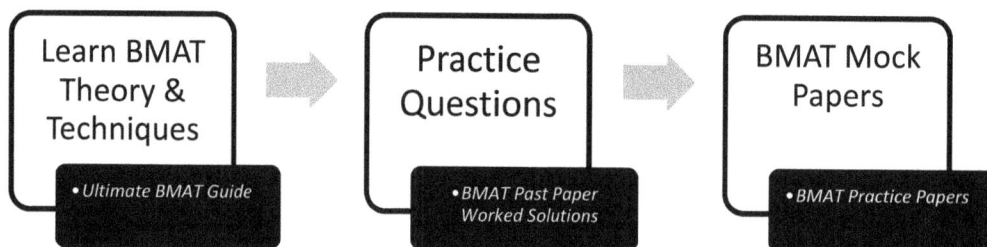

Learn BMAT Theory & Techniques		Practice Questions		BMAT Mock Papers
•Ultimate BMAT Guide	➡	•BMAT Past Paper Worked Solutions	➡	•BMAT Practice Papers

Scoring Tables

Use these to keep a record of your scores from past papers – you can then easily see which paper you should attempt next (always the one with the lowest score).

SECTION 1	1st Attempt	2nd Attempt	3rd Attempt
2003			
2004			
2005			
2006			
2007			
2008			
2009			
2010			
2011			
2012			
2013			
2014			
2015			
2016			
2017			

SECTION 2	1st Attempt	2nd Attempt	3rd Attempt
2003			
2004			
2005			
2006			
2007			
2008			
2009			
2010			
2011			
2012			
2013			
2014			
2015			
2016			
2017			

Section 3 will be much harder to mark with past papers due to the lack of example model answers to gauge yourself against. The *BMAT Past Paper Worked Solutions* book has detailed essay plans for every past paper. You can get a free copy by flicking to the back of this book.

And the same again here but with our mocks instead.

	SECTION 1	1st Attempt	2nd Attempt	3rd Attempt
olume One				
	Mock C			
olume Two				
	Mock F			
	Mock G			

	SECTION 2	1st Attempt	2nd Attempt	3rd Attempt
olume One				
	Mock D			
olume Two				
	Mock G			

Fortunately for our mock papers our tutors have compiled model answers for you to compare your essays against! If you're repeating a mock paper, its best to attempt a different essay title to give yourself maximum experience with the various styles of BMAT essays.

Volume One	Mock A	
	Mock D	
Volume Two		
	Mock H	

Remember! You can get a free copy of Volume 1 (Papers A to D) of *BMAT Practice Papers* by flicking to he back of this book.

MOCK PAPER E

Section 1

Question 1:

In regions of a comparatively low altitude many birds, as is well known, fly to the far North to find the proper climatic conditions in which to rear their broods and spend their summer vacation, some of them going to the subarctic provinces and others beyond. How different among the sublime heights of the Rockies! Here they are required to make a journey of only a few miles, say from five to one hundred or slightly more, according to the locality selected, up the defiles and canons or over the ridges, to find the conditions as to temperature, food, nesting sites, etc., that are precisely to their taste.

Which of the following statement can be reliably concluded from the above passage?
A) A journey of 100 miles is too far for these birds to travel for food.
B) Rearing their young is the most important part of these birds' lives.
C) These birds fly north as all their needs are in a localised area.
D) Nesting in the Rockies keeps the birds away from predators.
E) The birds struggle to survive in the harsh cold temperatures further north.

Question 2:

Three ladies X, Y and Z marry three men A, B and C. X is married to A, Y is not married to an engineer, Z is not married to a doctor, C is not a doctor and A is a lawyer.

Which of the following statements is correct?
A) Y is married to C, who is an engineer.
B) Z is married to C, who is a doctor.
C) X is married to a doctor.
D) None of the statements is correct.
E) All three statements are correct.

Question 3:

The medical scientific establishment has a long established system for naming body parts and medical phenomena. This system is based upon ease of understanding, such that a body part, or a process of the body, is named based on its clinical relevance. This means that features are named in a way which will help doctors understand and explain to patients what the body part is, or what is wrong with it in the case of a disease. However, this poses significant problems for scientific medical research. Often, the most important features of a body part from a scientific point of view are not the most clinically important features, leading to confusion within the scientific literature, as medical researchers misunderstand the purpose of a discussion, due to confusing nomenclature. Whilst it is important for doctors to be able to explain things clearly to patients, it is relatively easy for this to happen in spite of confusing nomenclature, whereas confusing names cause serious problems in the scientific world. Thus, the naming system for medical features should be edited, to reflect the scientifically important features of body parts, rather than the clinically important ones.

Which of the following best illustrates the main conclusion of this passage?
A) The naming system based on clinically important features causes problems in scientific literature.
B) Changing the naming system would allow faster progress to be made in scientific medical research.
C) The naming system should be changed to reflect the features of body parts which are most important scientifically.
D) The current naming system is sufficient and should not be changed to help lazy scientists who cannot be bothered to do fact-checking.
E) It is more important to have good doctor-patient relations than good progress in scientific research.

Question 4:

It is well established that modern humans evolved in Africa, around 2 million years ago, and that the first humans were mainly hunter-gatherers, living off hunted meat and plant foods collected from their environment. However, this poses an interesting question. Humans are relatively weak, small, feeble creatures, and around 2 million years ago most wildlife in Africa consisted of large, powerful creatures. Thus, it is unclear how humans were able to hunt successfully, and obtain meat for food. One theory is that humans are well-built for long-distance running, largely thanks to our ability to control our temperature via sweating.

This theory reasons that humans were able to pursue animals such as antelope, which run when challenged, and were able to keep on running until the antelope collapsed through heat exhaustion. Meanwhile, the humans were kept cool via sweating, and were able to then go in and butcher the defenceless antelope.

Recent evidence has emerged supporting this theory, showing that human feet are well-developed for long-distance running, with fleshy areas in the correct orientation to absorb the impact without causing joint damage, and a heart well evolved to keep pumping at a moderately fast pace for long periods. With the emergence of this powerful new evidence, we should accept this theory, known as "the persistence running theory" as true.

Which of the following identifies a flaw in this argument?
A) The emergence of evidence in support of the persistence running theory does not mean that this theory is true.
B) There is little evidence that the human body is well setup for long-distance running.
C) It has neglected to consider other theories for how humans obtained meat during their early evolution.
D) There are numerous issues with the theory of persistence running, but many of these have been resolved thanks to the new evidence that has emerged.
E) It has not considered evidence that humans evolved in Europe, where there are smaller animals which humans may have easily been able to tackle.

Question 5:

Sam needs to measure out exactly 4 litres of water into a tank. He has two pieces of equipment – a bucket that holds 5 litres and a one that holds 3 litres, with no intermediate markings.

Is it possible to measure out 4 litres? If so, how much water is needed in total in order to measure the 4 litres?

A) 4 litres

B) 7 litres

C) 8 litres

D) 10 litres

E) Not possible with this equipment

Question 6:

"A librarian is sorting books into their correct locations. All history books belong to the right of all science books. Science books are divided into five locations: engineering, biology, chemistry, physics and mathematics (in an uninterrupted order from right to left). Art books are located to the right of mathematics between engineering and sport, and sport books between art and history. Literature books are to the right of art books."

What can be certainly said about the location of literature books?

F) They are located between art and history books
G) They are located to the left of history books
H) They are located between mathematics and art
I) They are located to the right of engineering
J) They are not located to the left of sport

Question 7:

"Many people choose not to buy brand new cars, as buying brand new has significant disadvantages. Most importantly, a car's value drops substantially the moment it is first driven on the road. Even though a car is virtually unchanged by these first few miles, the potential resale value is significantly reduced. Therefore it is better to buy second hand cars, as their value does not drop so much immediately after purchase."

Which of the following best represents the main conclusion of this passage?

A) There are many equal reasons to avoid buying brand new cars
B) Cars that have driven lots of miles should be avoided
C) The rapid loss of value of new cars makes buying second-hand a wise choice
D) Second hand cars are at least as good as new ones
E) New cars should not be driven to ensure they keep their resale value

Question 8:

James is a wine dealer specialising in French wine. From his original stock of 2,000 bottles in one cellar, he sells 10% to one customer and 20% of the remaining wine to another customer. He makes £11,200 profit from the two transactions combined. What is the average profit per bottle?

A) £18   B) £20   C) £22   D) £24   E) £26

Question 9:

"Many good quality pieces of old furniture are considered 'timeless' – they are used and enjoyed by many people today, and this is expected to continue for many generations to come. However, most of this furniture dates back to previous eras, and modern furniture does not fall under the 'timeless' category of being enjoyed for many years to come."

Which of the following is the main flaw in the argument?
A) There may be many factors which make furniture good
B) There used to be more furniture makers than today
C) No evidence is given to tell us old furniture is better than new
D) Old furniture is desirable for other reasons than its quality
E) We cannot yet tell whether new furniture will become 'timeless'

Question 10:
"Red wine is thought to be much healthier than beer because it contains many antioxidants, which have been shown to be beneficial to health. Many red wines are produced in Southern France and Italy, therefore it is no surprise that residents there have a greater life expectancy than in the UK and Germany, which are predominantly beer producing countries."

Which of the following is an assumption of the above argument?

A) Italian people drink red wine
B) Antioxidants are beneficial for health
C) British people prefer beer to red wine
D) Beer is not produced in Italy
E) Italian life expectancy is greater than in the UK

Question 11:
Hannah, Jane and Tom are travelling to London to see a musical. Hannah catches the train at 1430. Jane leaves at the same time as Hannah, but catches a bus which takes 40% longer then Hannah's train. Tom also takes a train, and the journey time is 10 minutes less then Hannah's journey, but he leaves 45 minutes after Jane leaves. He arrives in London at 1620.

At what time will Jane arrive in London?

A) 1545   B) 1600   C) 1615   D) 1700   E) 1715

Question 12:
At a show, there are two different ticket prices for different seats. The cost is £10 for a standard seat, and £16 for a premium view seat. The total revenue from a show is £6,600, and the total attendance was 600.

How many premium view seats were purchased?

A) 60   B) 100   C) 140   D) 180   E) 240

Question 13:
The moon orbits the Earth once every 28 days. Between 20th January and 23rd May inclusive, how many degrees has the Moon turned through? This is not a leap year.

A) 1540°   B) 1560°   C) 1580°   D) 1600°   E) 1620°

Question 14:
Drama academies are special schools students can go to in order to learn performing arts. These schools are only available to the most skilled young performers, and aim to give students the best training in the arts, whilst still covering mainstream academic subjects. However, many parents are reluctant for their children to attend such academies, as they feel the academic teaching will be worse than at a standard school.

Which of the following, if true, would most weaken the above argument?

A) Most top actors attended a drama academy as children
B) There is as much time dedicated to academic work in drama academies as there is in normal schools
C) The academic work comprises a greater proportion of the study time than drama related activities
D) Most children are keen to attend a drama academy if given the opportunity
E) 80% of students at drama academies attain higher than average GCSE scores

Question 15:

Anil and Suresh both leave point A at the same time. Anil travels 5km East then 10km North. Anil then travels a further 1km North before heading 3km West. Suresh travels East for 2km less than Anil's total journey distance. He then heads 13km North, before pausing and travelling back 2km South. How far, as the crow flies, are the two men now apart?

A) 11km   B) 12km   C) 13km   D) 15km   E) 17km

Question 16:

Building foundations are covered by 14cm of concrete. A builder thinks this is too thick, and grinds down the concrete by an amount three times the thickness of the concrete which he eventually leaves.

What is the remaining thickness of concrete?

A) 1.5cm   B) 2.0cm   C) 2.5cm   D) 3.0cm   E) 3.5cm

Question 17:

Chris leaves his house to go and visit Laura, who lives 3 miles away. He leaves at 1730 and walks at 4mph towards Laura's house, stopping for one 5-minute to chat to a friend. Meanwhile Sarah also wants to visit Laura. She sets off from her house 6 miles away at 1810, driving in her car and averaging a speed of 24mph.

Who reaches the house first and with how long do they wait for the other person?
A) Chris, and waits 5 mins for Sarah   D) Sarah, and waits 10 mins for Chris
B) Chris, and waits 10 mins for Sarah   E) They both arrive at the same time
C) Sarah, and waits 5 mins for Chris

Question 18:

"Illegal film and music downloads have increased greatly in recent years. This causes significant harm to the relevant industries. Many people justify this to themselves by telling themselves they are only diverting money away from wealthy and successful singers and actors, who do not need any more money anyway. But in reality, illegal downloads are deeply harming the music industry, making many studio workers redundant and making it difficult for less famous performers to make a living."

Which of the following best summarises the conclusion of this argument?
A) Unemployment is a problem in the music industry
B) Taking profits away from successful musicians does more harm than good
C) Studio workers are most affected by illegal downloads
D) Illegal downloads cause more harm than people often think
E) Buying music legally helps keep the music industry productive

Question 19:

"40,000 litres of water will extinguish two typical house fires. 70,000 litres of water will extinguish two house fires and three garden fires. There is no surplus water"

Which statement is **NOT** true?

A) A garden fire can be extinguished with 12,000 litres, with water to spare.
B) 20,000 litres is sufficient to extinguish a normal house fire.
C) A garden fire requires only half as much water to extinguish as a house fire.
D) Two house and four garden fires will need 80,000 litres to extinguish.
E) Three house and ten garden fires will need 140,000 litres to extinguish.

Question 20:

A car travels at 20ms^{-1} for 30 seconds. It then accelerates at a constant rate of 2ms^{-2} for 5 seconds, then proceeds at the new speed for 20 seconds before braking with constant deceleration of 3ms^{-2} to a stop. What distance is covered in total?

A) 1325m   B) 1350m   C) 1375m   D) 1425m   E) 1475m

Question 21:

 "Plans are in place to install antennas underground, so that users of underground trains will be able to pick up mobile reception. There are, as usual, winners and losers from this policy. Supporters of the policy argue that it will lead to an increase in workforce productivity and increase convenience in day-to-day life. Critics respond by saying that it will lead to an annoying environment whilst travelling, it will facilitate the ease of conducting a terrorist threat and it will decrease levels of sociability. The latter camp seems to have the greatest support and so a re-consideration of the policy is urged."

Which of the following **best** summarises the conclusion of this passage?

A) The disadvantages of installing underground antennas outweigh the benefits
B) The cost of the scheme is likely to be prohibitive
C) The policy must be dropped, since a majority does not want it
D) More people don't want this scheme than do want it
E) A detailed consultation process should take place

Question 22:

"Ecosystems in the oceans are changing. Recently, restrictions on fishing have been imposed to tackle the decline in fish populations. As a result, farm fishing and the price of fish have increased, whilst the seas recover. It is hoped that these changes will lead to a brighter future for all."

Which of the following are **TWO** assumptions of this argument?

A) People will still buy farmed fish at a higher price
B) The population of wild fish can recover
C) Fishermen will benefit from working on this scheme
D) Ecosystems have been altered as a result of climate change
E) Heavy sea fishing is to blame for the changes in the ecosystem

Question 23:

Brian is tossing a coin. He tosses the coin 5 times. What is the probability of tossing exactly 2 heads?

A) $^{1}/_{16}$ B) $^{5}/_{32}$ C) $^{4}/_{16}$ D) $^{5}/_{16}$ E) $^{7}/_{16}$

Question 24:

The amount of a cleaning powder to be added to a bucket of water is determined by the volume of water, such that exactly 40g is added to each litre. A bucket contains 5 litres of water, and is required to have cleaning powder added. However, the markings on the bucket are only accurate to the nearest 2%. Calculate the difference between the maximum and minimum amounts of cleaning powder which might be required to be added to make up the solution correctly.

A) 4g   B) 6g   C) 8g   D) 12g   E) 20g

Question 25:

International telephone calls are charged at a rate per minute. For a call between two European countries, the rate is 22p per minute off-peak and 32p per minute at peak hours, rounded up to the nearest whole minute. In addition, there is a connection fee of 18p for every call.

What is the cost of an off-peak call from France to Germany, lasting 1.4 hours?

A) £18.48   B) £18.66   C) £26.88   D) £27.06   E) £30.98

Question 26:

"UV radiation is harmful to the skin, and can lead to the development of skin cancers. Despite this, many people sunbathe and use tanning salons, exposing themselves to dangerous radiation. If people took more sensible decisions about their health, many serious diseases, such as skin cancers, could be avoided."

What is the main conclusion of this passage?

A) UV radiation is harmful to the skin
B) Many people like to get tanned, despite the risks
C) People do not always consider the health risks of choices they make
D) Skin cancer is a serious disease
E) Sunbathing is risky, and people should avoid it

Question 27:

Jim washes windows for pocket money. Washing a window takes two minutes. Between one house and the next, it takes Jim 15 minutes to pack up, walk to the next house and get ready to start washing again. Each resident pays Jim £3 per house, regardless of how many windows the house has. In one day, Jim washes 8 houses, with an average of 11 windows per house.

What is his equivalent hourly pay rate?

A) £4.38   B) £4.86   C) £5.12   D) £5.62   E) £6.12

Question 28:

"Bottled water is becomingly increasingly popular, but it is hard to see why. Bottled water costs many hundreds of times more than a virtually identical product from the tap, and bears a significant environmental cost of transportation. Those who argue in favour of bottled water may point out that the flavour is slightly better – but would you pay 300 times the price for a car with just a few added features?"
Which of the following, if true, would most weaken the above argument?

A) Bottled water has many health benefits in addition to tasting nicer
B) Bottled water does not taste any different to tap water
C) The cost of transportation is only a fraction of the costs associated with bottling and selling water
D) Some people do buy very expensive cars
E) Buying bottled water supports a big industry, providing many jobs to people

Question 29:

"There are no marathon runners that aren't skinny, nor no cyclists that aren't marathon runners."
Which of the following **must** be true?

A) Cyclists do not run marathons
B) Cyclists are all skinny
C) Any skinny person is also a cyclist

D) Marathon runners must all be cyclists
E) All of the above

Question 30:

"Langham is East of Hadleigh but West of Frampton. Oakton is midway between Langham and Stour. Frampton is West of Stour. Manley is not East of Langham."
Which of the following **cannot** be concluded?

A) Oakton is East of Langham and Hadleigh.
B) Frampton is West of Stour and East of Manley.
C) Stour is East of Hadleigh and Langham.
D) Oakton is East of Langham and West of Frampton
E) Manley is West of Oakton and West of Frampton.

Question 31:

A pot of paint gives sufficient paint to cover $12m^2$ of wall area. The inner surface of a planetarium must be painted. The planetarium consists of a hemispheric dome of internal diameter 14 metres. How many pots of paint are required to give the dome two full coats of paint? [Assume $\pi=3$]

A) 25   B) 36   C) 49   D) 64   E) 98

Question 32:

A planetarium has just been painted as in **31**, above. Assuming each pot of paint is 2 litres, and that the solid component of the paint is 40%, calculate the percentage decrease in the volume of the planetarium, due to the painting.

A) 0.0029%   B) 0.0057%   C) 0.029%   D) 0.057%   E) 2.86%

END OF SECTION

Section 2

Question 1:
The buoyancy force of an object is the produce of its volume, density and the gravitational constant, g. A boat weighing 600 kg with a density of $1000kgm^{-3}$ and hull volume of 950 litres is placed in a lake. What is the minimum mass that, if added to the boat, will cause it to sink? Use $g = 10ms^{-1}$.

A) 3.55 kg

B) 35 kg

C) 350 kg

D) 355 kg

E) 3,550 kg

F) None, the boat has already sunk

Question 2:
Which of the following below is **NOT** an example of an oxidation reaction?

A) $Li^+ + H_2O \rightarrow Li^+ + OH^- + \frac{1}{2}H_2$

B) $N_2 \rightarrow 2N^+ + 2e^-$

C) $2CH_4 + 2O_2 \rightarrow 2CH_2O + 2H_2O$

D) $2N_2 + O_2 \rightarrow 2N_2O$

E) $I_2 + 2e^- \rightarrow 2I^-$

F) All of the above are oxidation reactions

Question 3:
An investment of £500 is made in a compound interest account. At the end of 3 years the balance reads £1687.50. What is the interest rate?

A) 20%   B) 35%   C) 50%   D) 65%   E) 80%

Question 4:
Mr Khan fires a bullet at a speed of 310 ms^{-1} from a height of 1.93m parallel to the floor. Mr Weeks drops an identical bullet from the same height.

What is the time difference between the bullets first making contact with the floor?[Assume that there is negligible air resistance; $g= 10$ ms^{-2}]

A) 0 s

B) 0.2 s

C) 1.93 s

D) 2.1 s

E) More information is needed

Question 5:
Rupert plays one game of tennis and one game of squash.
The probability that he will win the tennis game is 3/4
The probability that he will win the squash game is 1/3
What is the probability that he will win one game only?

A) 3/12   B) 7/12   C) 4/5   D) 13/12   E) 7/6

Question 6:
Jane is one mile into a marathon. Which of the following statements is **NOT** true, relative to before she started?

A) Blood flow to the skin is increased

B) Blood flow to the muscles is increased

C) Blood flow to the gut is decreased

D) Blood flow to the kidneys is decreased

E) Cardiac Output Increases

F) None of the above

Question 7:
Balance the following chemical equation. What is the value of **x**?

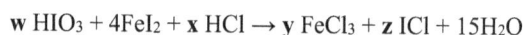

$$\textbf{w}\ HIO_3 + 4FeI_2 + \textbf{x}\ HCl \rightarrow \textbf{y}\ FeCl_3 + \textbf{z}\ ICl + 15H_2O$$

A) 4   B) 5   C) 9   D) 15   E) 22   F) 25

Question 8:
A newly discovered species of beetle is found to have 29.6% Adenine (A) bases in its genome. What is the percentage of Cytosine (C) bases in the beetle's DNA?

A) 20.4%
B) 29.6%
C) 40.8%

D) 59.2%
E) 70.6%
F) More information is required

Question 9:
Study the following diagram of the human heart. What is true about structure **A**?

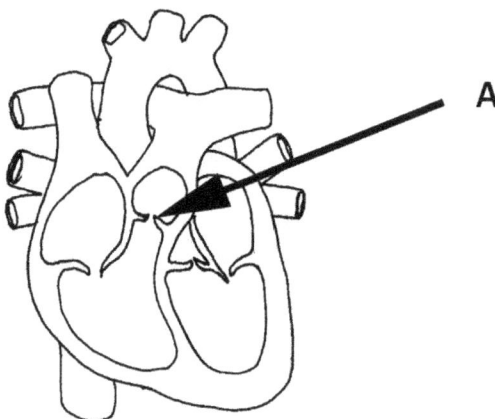

A) It is closed during systole
B) It prevents blood flowing into the left ventricle during systole
C) It prevents blood flowing into the right ventricle during systole
D) It prevents blood flowing into the left ventricle during diastole
E) It opens due to left ventricular pressure being greater than aortic pressure.
F) It is open when the right ventricle is emptying

Question 10:
Carbon monoxide binds irreversibly to the oxygen binding site of haemoglobin. Which of the following statements is true regarding carbon monoxide poisoning?

A) Carbon monoxide poisoning has no serious consequences
B) Haemoglobin is heavier, as both oxygen and carbon monoxide bind to it
C) Affected individuals have a raised heart rate
D) The CO_2 carrying capacity of the blood is decreased
E) The O_2 carrying capacity of the blood is unchanged as it dissolves in the plasma instead

Question 11:

A crane is 40 m tall. The lifting arm is 5m long and the counterbalance arm is 2m long. The beam joining the two weighs 350kg, and is of uniform thickness. The lifting arm lifts a 2000 kg mass. What counterbalance mass is required to balance exactly around the centre point? Use $g = 10$ ms^{-2}.

A) 4,220 kg   C) 5,013 kg   E) 10,525 kg
B) 4,820 kg   D) 5,263 kg

Question 12:

For Christmas, Mr James decorates his house with 20 strings of 150 bulbs each. Each 150-bulb string of lights is rated at 50 Watts. Mr James turns the lights on at 8pm and off at 6am each night. The lights are used for 20 days in total.

If 100 kJ of energy costs 2p, how much is the total cost Mr James has to pay?

A) £2160.00   B) £144.00   C) £14.40   D) £0.72   E) £0.24

Question 13:

Calculate the perimeter of a regular polygon each interior angle is 150° and each side is 15 cm.

A) 75 cm   D) 225 cm   F) More information is
B) 150 cm   E) 1,500 cm   needed.
C) 180 cm

Question 14:

The diagram shown below depicts an electrical circuit with multiple resistors, each with equal resistance, Z. The total resistance between A and B is 22 MΩ. Calculate the value of Z.

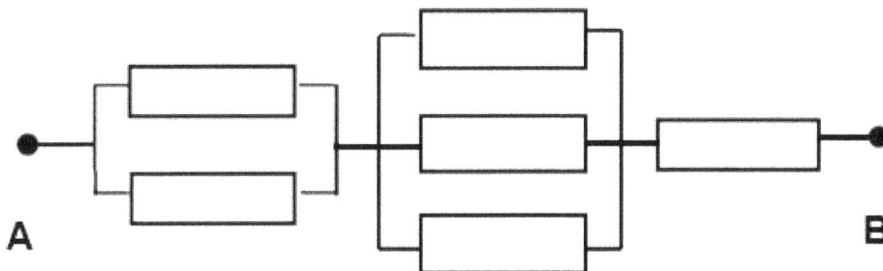

A) 3.33 MΩ   B) 4.33 MΩ   C) 7.33 MΩ   D) 11 MΩ   E) 12 MΩ

Question 15:

A cylindrical candle of diameter 4cm burns steadily at a rate of 1cm per hour. Assuming the candle is composed entirely of paraffin wax ($C_{24}H_{52}$) of density 900 kgm^{-3} and undergoes complete combustion, how much energy is transferred in 30 minutes? You may assume the molar combustion energy is 11,000 kJmol^{-1}, and that $\pi=3$.

A) 140,000J   C) 185,000J   E) 215,000J
B) 175,000J   D) 200,500J   F) 348,000J

Question 16:

A different candle to that in question **15** is used to heat a bucket of water. The candle burns for 45 minutes, releasing 250KJ of energy as heat. It is used to heat a 2 litre bucket of water at 25°C.

Assuming the bucket is completely insulated, what is the water temperature after 45 minutes? (For reference: One calorie heats one cm^3 of water by one degree Celsius, 1kCal = 4,200J).

A) 35°C
B) 45°C

C) 55°C
D) 65°C

E) 75°C
F) 85°C

Question 17:

A person responds to the starting gun of a race and begins to run. Place the following order of events in the most likely chronological sequence. Which option is a correct sequence?

1 Blood CO_2 increases

2 The eardrum vibrates to the sound

3 Impulses travel along motor neurones

4 Impulses travel along sensory neurones

5 Impulses travel along relay neurones

6 Quadriceps muscles contract

7 Glycogen is converted into glucose

8 Creatine phosphate rapidly re-phosphorylates ADP

A) $2 \rightarrow 5 \rightarrow 4 \rightarrow 3 \rightarrow 6 \rightarrow 7$
B) $2 \rightarrow 4 \rightarrow 3 \rightarrow 8 \rightarrow 6 \rightarrow 1$
C) $2 \rightarrow 3 \rightarrow 4 \rightarrow 6 \rightarrow 7 \rightarrow 1$

D) $2 \rightarrow 4 \rightarrow 3 \rightarrow 1 \rightarrow 6 \rightarrow 7$
E) $2 \rightarrow 4 \rightarrow 3 \rightarrow 6 \rightarrow 8 \rightarrow 7$

Question 18:

On analysis, an organic substance is found to contain 41.4% Carbon, 55.2% Oxygen and 3.45% Hydrogen by mass. Which of the following could be the chemical formula of this substance?

A) $C_3O_3H_6$
B) $C_3O_3H_{12}$

C) $C_4O_2H_4$
D) $C_4O_4H_4$

E) $C_4O_2H_8$
F) More information needed

Question 19:

Simplify and solve: (e - a) (e + b) (e – c) (e + d)…(e - z)?

A) 0
B) e^{26}

C) e^{26} (a-b+c-d...+z)
D) e^{26} (a+b-c+d...-z)

E) e^{26} (abcd...z)
F) None of the above.

Question 20:

Which of the following best describes the events that occur during expiration?

A) The ribs move up and in; the diaphragm moves down.
B) The ribs move down and in; the diaphragm moves up.
C) The ribs move up and in; the diaphragm moves up.
D) The ribs move down and out; the diaphragm moves down.
E) The ribs move up and out; the diaphragm moves down.
F) The ribs move up and out; the diaphragm moves up.

Question 21:

Simplify fully: $1 + \left(3\sqrt{2} - 1\right)^2 + \left(3 + \sqrt{2}\right)^2$

A)   C)   E) 29
B)   D) 24   F) 31

Question 22:

200 cm^3 of a 1.8 moldm^{-3} solution of sodium nitrate (NaNO$_3$) is used in a chemical reaction. How many moles of sodium nitrate is this?

A) 0.09 mol   B) 0.36 mol   C) 9.00 mol   D) 36.0 mol   E) 360 mol

Question 23:

A tourist at Victoria Falls accidentally drops her 400g camera. It falls 125 metres into the water below. Assuming resistive forces to be zero and g = 10ms^{-1}, what is the momentum of the camera the instant before it strikes the water? [Momentum = mass x velocity]

A) 4 kgms^{-1} C) 16 kgms^{-1} E) 50 kgms^{-1}
B) 13 kgms^{-1} D) 20 kgms^{-1} F) 20,000 kgms^{-1}

Question 24:

Antibiotics can have serious side effects such as liver failure and renal failure. Therefore, scientists are always trying to develop antibiotics to minimise these effects by targeting specific cellular components. Which of these cellular components offers the best way to treat infections and minimise side effects?

A) Mitochondrion   C) Nucleic acid   E) Flagellum
B) Cell membrane   D) Cytoskeleton

Question 25:

A is a group 3 element and B is a group 6 element. Which row best describes what happens to A when it reacts with B?

	Electrons are	Size of Atom
A)	Gained	Increases
B)	Gained	Decreases
C)	Gained	Unchanged
D)	Lost	Increases
E)	Lost	Decreases
F)	Lost	Unchanged

Question 26:

Each vertex of a square lies directly on the edge of a circle with a radius of 1cm. Calculate the area of the circle that is not occupied by the square. Use $\pi = 3$.

A) 0.25cm^2 C) 0.75cm^2 E) 1.25cm^2
B) 0.5cm^2 D) 1.0cm^2 F) 1.5cm^2

Question 27:

A funicular railway like the one illustrated lifts a full carriage weighing 3600kg up an incline. The distance travelled is 200m, and the vertical ascent, **v**, is 80m. Ten passengers weighing an average of 72kg disembark, then the carriage descends. As a result of efficient design, the energy from the descent is stored to drive the next ascent.

Assuming the same load of 10 passengers then enters the car, how powerful an engine is required to move the carriage at 4ms^{-1}?

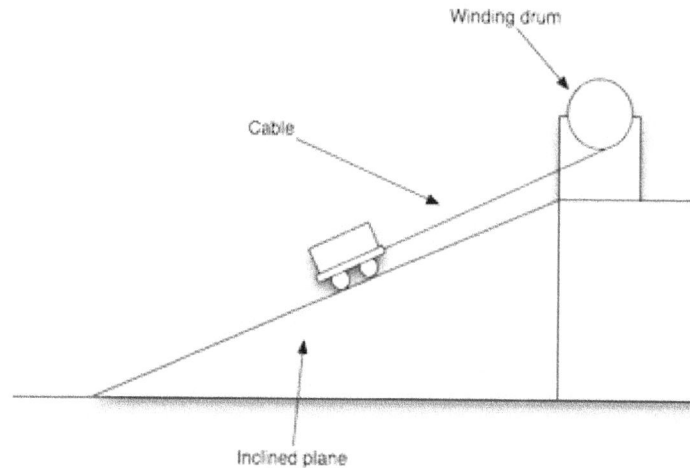

A) 9.2 kW   B) 11.5 kW   C) 28.8 kW   D) 46.1 kW   E) 57.6 kW

END OF SECTION

Section 3

1)   *'Doctors know best and should decide which treatment a patient receives'*

Explain what this statement alludes to. Argue to the contrary that patients know best and should be able to choose their management plan. To what extent do you agree with this statement?

2)   *'World peace will be achieved in the future'*

Explain what this statement means. Argue to the contrary, that world peace will never be achieved. To what extent, if any, do you agree with the statement?

3)   *'Medicine is a science; not an art'*

Explain what this statement means. Argue to the contrary that medicine is in fact an art using examples to illustrate your answer. To what extent, if any, is medicine a science?

4)   *'People should live healthier lives to reduce the financial burden of healthcare to the taxpayer.'*

Explain what this statement means. Argue to the contrary. To what extent do you agree with the statement?

END OF PAPER

MOCK PAPER F

Section 1

Question 1:

Every year, there are tens of thousands of motor crashes, causing a serious number of fatalities. Indeed, this represents the leading cause of death in the UK that is not a disease. In spite of this horrendous statistic, there are still thousands of uninsured drivers. The government is under moral obligation to clamp down on uninsured drivers, to reduce the incidence of such crashes. That they have not acted is arguably the most outrageous failing of the present government.

Which of the following is the best statement of a **flaw** in this passage?

A) It has made unsupported claims that the government's failure to act is morally outrageous.
B) It has not provided any evidence to support its claims that motor crashes are the leading cause of death in the UK outside of diseases.
C) Even if motor crashes were prevented, it would not save lives of people who die from other causes.
D) It has implied that lack of insurance is related to the incidence of motor crashes.
E) It has fabricated an obligation on the government's part to intervene and reduce the numbers of uninsured drivers.

Question 2:

Several years ago the Brazilian government held a referendum of the populace, to decide whether they should enact a law banning the ownership of guns. The Brazilian people voted strongly against this proposal. When asked why this had happened, one commentator said he believed the reason was that 90% of criminals who use guns to commit crimes buy their weapons on the black market, illegally. Thus, if Brazil were to ban the legal sale of guns, this would remove the ability of law-abiding citizens to purchase protection, whilst doing little to remove weapons from the hands of criminals.

Some commentators have pointed to this statistic, and claimed that the UK should also legalise guns, to allow citizens to protect themselves. However, in the UK the black market for weapons is not as widespread as in Brazil. Most people in the UK have little reason to fear gun attacks, and legalising the sale of guns would simply make it much easier for criminals to acquire weapons.

Which of the following best expresses the main conclusion of this passage?

A) The UK should not follow Brazil's lead on gun legislation.
B) Efforts to reduce gun ownership should focus on the black market.
C) Violent crime is a more pressing concern in Brazil than the UK.
D) Legalising the sale of guns in the UK would result in widespread ownership.
E) Criminals will always find a way to obtain firearms.

Question 3:

Hannah is buying tiles for her new bathroom. She wants to use the same tiles on the floor and all 4 walls and for all the walls to be completely tiled apart from the door. The bathroom is 2.4 metres high, 2 metres wide and 2 metres long, and the door is 2 metres high, 80cm wide and at the end of one of the 4 identical walls. The tiles she wants to use are 40cm x 40cm.
How many of these tiles does she need to tile the whole bathroom?

A) 110   B) 120   C) 135   D) 145   E) 150

Question 4:

Jane and Trevor are both travelling south, from York to London. Jane is driving, whilst Trevor is travelling by train. The speed limit on the roads between York and London is 70mph, whilst the train travels at 90mph. Thus, we should expect that Trevor will arrive first.

Which of the following would weaken this passage's conclusion?

A) The train takes a direct route, whilst the road from York to London goes through several major cities and zig-zags somewhat on its way down the country.
B) Trevor left before Jane.
C) Jane is a conscientious driver, who never exceeds the speed limit.
D) Trevor's train makes a lot of stops on the way, and spends several minutes at each stop waiting for new passengers to board.
E) Meanwhile, Raheem is making the same journey by plane, and will arrive before either Trevor or Jane.

Question 5:

A recipe for 20 cupcakes needs 200g of butter, 200g of sugar, 200g of flour and 4 eggs. Jeremy has two 250g packs of butter, a bag of 600g of sugar, a kilogram bag of flour and a pack of 12 eggs.

How many cupcakes can he make and how many eggs does he have left over?

A) 50, 2   B) 50, 3   C) 60, 0   D) 60, 2   E) 60, 3

Question 6:

ABC taxis charges a rate of 15p per minute, plus £4. XYZ taxis charges a rate of £4 plus 30p per mile. I live 6 miles from the station.

What would the taxi's average speed have to be on my journey home from the station for the two taxi firms to charge exactly the same fare?

A) 25   B) 30   C) 45   D) 55   E) 60

Question 7:

King Arthur has been issued a challenge by Mordac, his nephew who rules the adjacent Kingdom. Mordac has challenged King Arthur to select a knight to complete a series of challenging obstacles, battling a number of dark creatures along the way, in a test known as the Adzol. The King's squire reports that there are tales told by the elders of the court meaning that only a knight with tremendous courage will succeed in Adzol, and all others will fail. He therefore suggests that Arthur should select Lancelot, the most courageous of all Arthur's Knights. The squire argues that due to what the Elders have said, Lancelot will succeed in the task, but all others will fail.

Which of the following is **NOT** an assumption in the squire's reasoning?

A) Lancelot has sufficient courage to succeed in the Adzol.
B) No other knights in Arthur's command also have tremendous courage, so will all fail Adzol.
C) Great courage is required to be successful in the Adzol.
D) The tales told by the elders of the court are correct.
E) None of the above – they are all assumptions.

Question 8:

A historian is examining a recently excavated hall beneath a medieval castle. She finds that there are a series of arch-shaped gaps along one length of the wall, surrounded by a different pattern of bricks to that seen elsewhere in the walls. These are found to represent where windows where once located, looking out onto one side of the castle. However, the site is now underground. Underground halls in castles never contain windows, so the historian reasons that this hall must once have been located above the ground. Therefore, the ground level must have changed since this castle was built.

Which of the following represents the main conclusion of this passage?

A) Windows are never found in underground halls.
B) Arch-shaped gaps always indicate that windows were once present.
C) It is unexpected for windows to be found in halls in castles.
D) The hall was once located above ground.
E) The ground level must have changed since this hall was built.

Question 9:

Adam's grandmother has sent him to the shop to buy bread rolls. Usually, bread rolls are 30p for a pack of 6 and so his grandmother has given him the exact amount to buy a certain number of bread rolls. However, today there is a special offer whereby if you buy 3 or more packs of rolls, the price per roll is reduced by 1p. He can now buy 1 more pack than before and get no change.
How many bread rolls was he originally supposed to buying?

A) 4 B) 5 C) 6 D) 24 E) 30

Question 10:

The England men's cricket team have recently been knocked out of the world cup after a very poor performance that saw them eliminated at the group stage, managing only 1 win and losing against teams well below them in the rankings. The board of English cricket is sitting down to discuss why the team's performance was so poor, and what can be done to ensure that future world cups have a more positive outcome. The chairman of the board says that the current crop of players is not good enough, and that the team's performance should improve soon, as more able players come through the ranks in the county teams, so no action is needed.

However, the sporting director takes a different view, saying that England have not gone further than the group stage of any cricket world cup for the last 25 years, during which time numerous players have come and gone from the team. The sporting director argues that this long period of poor performance indicates that there is a problem with English cricket, meaning that not enough talented players are being produced in the country. He argues that therefore, steps should be taken to reform English cricket to actively foster the development of more talented players.

Which of the following, if true, would most strengthen the sporting director's argument?

A) The English cricket team is regarded as one of the best in the world, with some of the most talented players.
B) England have been steadily falling lower in the world cricket rankings for the last 25 years, due to poor performances across the board in various cricket competitions.
C) A skilled batsman, who was ranked as the 4th best player in the world, has recently retired from the England team. Now, there are no English cricket players in the top 10 of the world cricket player rankings, which is the first time this has happened in over 70 years.
D) Despite not performing well in world cups, England have performed well in other cricket competitions over the last 20 years.
E) Cricket was invented in England, so everybody expects that England should have a lot of good players in their team.

Question 11:

Karl is making cupcakes for a wedding. It takes him 25 minutes to prepare each batch of cakes. Only 12 can go in the oven at a time and each batch takes 20 minutes in the oven.

What is the latest time Karl can start if he needs to make 100 cupcakes by 4pm?

A) 11:55am   B) 12:20pm   C) 12:40pm   D) 13:20pm   E) 14:00pm

Question 12:

	Boys Absenteeism	Girls Absenteeism	Pupils on Roll	Average
Hazelwood Grammar	7%	Boys' School	300	7%
Heather Park Academy	5%	6%	1000	5.60%
Holland Wood Comprehensive	5%	6%	500	5.60%
Hurlington Academy	Girls' School		200	
Average		7%		

Some of the information is missing from the table above. What is the rate of girls' absenteeism at Hurlington Academy?

A) 6.5%   B) 7%   C) 9%   D) 11.5%   E) 13%

Question 13:

Up until the 20th century, all watches were made by hand, by watchmakers. Watchmaking is considered one of the most difficult and delicate of manufacturing skills, requiring immense patience, meticulous attention to detail and an extremely steady hand. However, due to the advent of more accurate technology, most watches are now produced by machines, and only a minority are made by hand, for specialist collectors. Thus, some watchmakers now work for the watch industry, and only perform *repairs* on watches that are initially produced by machines.

Which of the following *cannot* be reliably concluded from this passage?

A) Most watches are now produced by machines, not by hand.
B) Watchmaking is considered one of the most difficult of manufacturing skills
C) Most watchmakers now work for the watch industry, performing repairs on watches rather than producing new ones.
D) The advent of more accurate technology caused the situation today, where most watches are made by machines.
E) Some watches are now made by hand for specialist collectors.

Question 14:

Many vegetarians claim that they do not eat meat, poultry or fish because it is unethical to kill a sentient being. Most agree that this argument is logical. However, some Pescatarians have also used this argument, that they do not eat meat because they do not believe in killing sentient beings, but they are happy to eat fish. This argument is clearly illogical. There is powerful evidence that fish fulfil just as much of the criteria for being sentient as do most commonly eaten animals, such as chicken or pigs, but that all these animals lack certain criteria for being "sentient" that humans possess. Thus, pescatarians should either accept the killing of beings less sentient than humans, and thus be happy to eat meat and poultry, or they should not accept the killing of any partially sentient beings, and thus not be happy to eat fish.

Which of the following best illustrates the main **conclusion** of this passage?

A) The argument that it is unethical to eat meat due to not wishing to kill sentient beings but eating fish is acceptable is illogical.
B) Pescatarians cannot use logic.
C) Fish are just as sentient as chicken and pigs, and all these beings are less sentient than humans.
D) It is not unethical to eat meat, poultry or fish.
E) It is unethical to eat all forms of meat, including fish and poultry.

Question 15:
Recent research into cultural attitudes in British has revealed a striking hypocrisy. When asked whether foreign people travelling to British on holiday should learn some English, 60% of respondents answered yes. However, when asked if they would attempt to learn some of the language before travelling to a country which did not speak English, only 15% of the respondents answered yes. This is a shocking double-standard on the part of the British public, and is symptomatic of a deeper underlying issue that British people feel themselves superior to other cultures.

Which of the following can be reliably concluded from this passage?

A) 60% of people in Britain think that foreign people travelling to Britain for a holiday should learn English, but would not learn the language themselves when going on holiday to a country which did not speak English.
B) The British public do not feel that it is important to learn some of the language before travelling to a country which does not speak English.
C) There are numerous issues of racism amongst the British public, stemming from the fact they feel themselves superior to other cultures.
D) Less than 10% of the British public would attempt to learn some of the language before travelling to a country which did not speak English.
E) Some in Britain think that foreign people travelling to Britain for a holiday should learn English, but would not learn the language themselves when going on holiday to a country which did not speak English.

Question 16:
Harriet is a headmistress and she is making 400 information packs for the sixth form open evening. Each information pack needs to have 2 double sided sheets of A4 of general information about the school. She also needs to produce 50 A5 single sided sheets about each of the 30 A Level courses on offer. Single sided A5 costs £0.01 per sheet. Double sided costs twice as much as single sided. A4 printing costs 1.5 times as much as A5.

How much does she spend altogether on the printing?

A) £27   B) £31   C) £35   D) £39   E) £43

Question 17:

Kirkleatham Town football club are currently leading the league. One week they play a crucial match against Redcar Rovers, who are second placed. The points tally of the teams in the table means that if Kirkleatham Town win this game, they will win the league. Before the game, the manager of Kirkleatham Town says that Redcar Rovers are a tough opponent, and that if his team do not play with desire and commitment, they will not win the game. After the game, the manager is asked for comment on the game, and says he was pleased that his team played with so much desire, and showed high levels of commitment. Therefore, Kirkleatham will win the league.

Which of the following best illustrates a flaw in this passage?

A) It has assumed that Kirkleatham will not win the game if they do not play with desire and commitment.
B) It has assumed that if Kirkleatham play with desire and commitment, they will win the game.
C) It has assumed that Kirkleatham played with desire and commitment.
D) It has assumed that Redcar Rovers are a tough opponent, and that Kirkleatham will not be able to easily win the game.
E) It has assumed that if Kirkleatham win the match against Redcar Rovers, they will win the league.

Question 18:

Two councillors are considering planning proposals for a new housing estate, to be built on the edge of Bluedown Village. Councillor Johnson argues for a proposal to be built upon brownfield land, land which has previously been built on, rather than greenbelt land, which has not previously been built on. He argues that this will both lower the cost of building the estate, as the land would already have some underlying infrastructure and would not need as much preparation, and will ensure a minimal impact on wildlife around the area.

Which of the following would most weaken the councillor's argument?

A) Brownfield land is often not as appealing as greenbelt land visually, and it is likely that houses built on brownfield land will not sell for as high a price as houses built on greenbelt land.
B) An area of brownfield land on the edge of the village, originally built as an outdoor leisure complex, has since become run down, and ironically is now a haven for various types of rare newts, lizards and birds.
C) Much of the brownfield land around the edge of the village has undergone substantial underground development, with a good system of electricity cables, gas pipes and plumbing in place.
D) The village is surrounded by several greenbelt areas designated as areas of outstanding natural beauty, supporting an abundance of wildlife.
E) The village mayor, who has ultimate control over the planning proposal, agrees with councillor Johnson's argument. Thus, it is likely his recommendations will be followed

Question 19:

	Pool A	Pool B	Pool C	Pool D
1st	France	Argentina	England	South Africa
2nd	Holland	Mexico	Nigeria	Brazil
3rd	United States	Denmark	Germany	Japan
4th	India	Korea	Ghana	Algeria
5th	Australia	Switzerland	Portugal	Serbia
6th	Greece	New Zealand	Honduras	Uruguay
7th	Chile	Slovakia	Cameroon	Paraguay

The table above shows the final standings in the pool stages of a football competition. The top 2 teams from each pool progress into the quarterfinals. The fixtures for the quarterfinals are determined as follows:

QF1: Winners Pool A vs. Runner up Pool B

QF2: Winners Pool B vs. Runner up Pool C

QF3: Winners Pool C vs. Runner up Pool D

QF4: Winners Pool D vs. Runner up Pool A

The winners of QF1 then play the winners of QF3 in one semifinal, and the winners of QF2 and winners of QF4 play each other in the other semifinal. The winners of the semi-finals progress to the final.
Which of these teams could England play in the final?

A) Nigeria   B) France   C) Mexico   D) Denmark   E) Brazil

Question 20:
The pie chart shows the voting intentions of some constituents interviewed by a polling group, prior to an upcoming election.

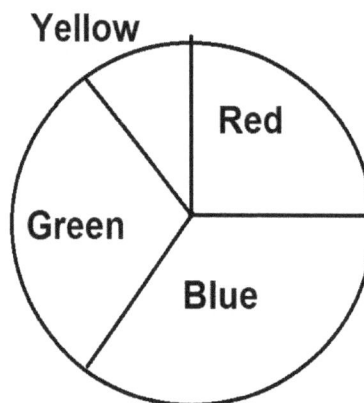

Yellow

Red

Green

Blue

How many times more people said their intention was to vote for the red party than the yellow party?

A) 2   B) 3   C) 4   D) 5   E) 6

Question 21:

A pizza takeaway is having a sale. If you spend £30 or more at full price, you can get 40% off.

Prices are as follows:

- Basic cheese and tomato pizza: £8 small, £10 large
- All other toppings are £1 each
- Sides are: Garlic bread £3, Potato wedges £2.50, Chips £1.50 and Dips £1 each

Ellie and Mike want to order a large pizza with mushrooms and ham, garlic bread, 2 portions of chips and a dip.

Which of these additional items can they order to minimise the amount they have to pay?

A) Small pizza with pineapple and onion

B) Large pizza with mushroom

C) Barbecue dip

D) 4 portions of potato wedges

E) Garlic bread

Question 22:

	Goals Scored	Goals Conceded
City	10	4
United	8	5
Rovers	1	10

The table above shows the goal scoring record of teams in a football tournament. Each team plays the other teams twice, once at home and once away. Here are the results of the first 4 matches:

➢ United 2 – 2 City

➢ Rovers 0 – 3 City

➢ City 2 – 1 Rovers

➢ Rovers 0 – 3 United

What were the results of the final two fixtures?

A) United 2 – 0 Rovers, City 0 – 0 United

B) United 1 – 0 Rovers, City 1 – 1 United

C) United 0 – 0 Rovers, City 2 – 1 United

D) United 1 – 0 Rovers, City 2 – 2 United

E) United 2 – 0 Rovers, City 3 – 1 United

Question 23:

The M1 Abrams tank is widely regarded as the most fearsome tank in the world. Highly advanced depleted uranium composite armour makes it difficult to damage from range, whilst a good top speed in excess of 50kmph and a large fuel capacity make it difficult to catch and contain the tank in an operational context. Whilst the tank does have weak spots that can be exploited at close range, a formidable 122m smoothbore gun as the main armament makes this an incredibly dangerous tactic for opposing tanks.

Country X is developing a new main battle tank to boost the prowess of their armoured formations, and have released a statement describing how they will implement next-generation armour into this new tank, to boost its defensive capacity. The government of country X believe this will allow their new tank to compete with the best tanks in the world. However, this view is mistaken. The M1 Abrams clearly demonstrates that a *combination* of different factors, including protection, manoeuvrability and firepower, are responsible for its status as the world's most formidable tank. Simply increasing the defensive capabilities of a tank is not sufficient. Thus, Country X's government is clearly incorrect in this matter.

Which of the following best illustrates the main conclusion of this passage?

A) Increasing the defensive capacity of a tank is not sufficient to make it equal to the best tanks in the world.
B) Multiple factors are required to make a tank equal to the best tanks in the world.
C) The new tank will not be as good as the M1 Abrams, as its defensive capacity will not be as good.
D) The view of Country X's government, that increasing the defensive capacity of a tank will make it equal to the best in the world, is clearly incorrect.
E) No tank is able to compete with the M1 Abrams, which will always be the world's most formidable tank.

Question 24:

The table below shows the balances of my bank accounts in pounds. Interest is paid at the end of the calendar year. My salary, which is the same every month, is paid into my current account on the 2nd of each month. All the money I have is in one or other of my bank accounts.

	Current Account	Savings	ISA
1st March	1300	5203	2941
1st April	3249	2948	2941
1st May	4398	9384	0
1st June	3948	8292	0

In which month did I spend the most money?

A) February
B) March
C) April
D) May
E) 2 or more months are the same

Question 25:

On Monday, my son developed a disease; no one else in the house has the disease. The doctor gave me some medicine and told me that everyone in the house who does not have the disease should also take half the dose. We need to take the medicine for 10 days, and the dosage is based on weight.

Weight	Dosage
Under 30kg	0.1ml per kg, 3 times a day
30kg – 60kg	0.2ml per kg, 4 times a day
60kg +	0.1ml per kg, 6 times a day

My son is 40 kg. I also have a daughter who is 20 kg. I am 75 kg and my husband is 80 kg. How many 200 ml bottles of medicine will we need for the whole 10 days?

A) 4   B) 5   C) 6   D) 7   E) 8

Question 26:

At Tina's nursery school, they have red, yellow or blue plastic cutlery. They have just enough forks and just enough knives for the 21 children there. There are the same number of forks as knives of each colour. Twice as many pieces of cutlery are yellow as blue. Half as many pieces of cutlery are red as blue. Tina takes a fork and a knife at random. What is the probability that she will get her favourite combination, a red fork and a yellow knife?

A) 4/49   B) 1/9   C) 36/49   D) 3/9   E) 3/49

Question 27:

The UK's taxation and public spending is horrendously flawed, with various immoral features. One example of such a flaw is the subsidy of public transport with money raised via taxation. According to recent research, public transport is only used by 65% of the population, and since there is no economic benefit stemming from a good public transport system, the other 35% of the population gets no benefit from public transport, but are still required to pay towards it via taxation. The system is in urgent need of reform, such that taxation is only used to support services and systems which are of benefit to everyone.

Which of the following is the best application of the principle used in this passage?

A) Only 48% of the population have ever visited an art gallery, so public funds should not be used to subsidise art galleries, as not all the population use it.
B) Primary and Secondary education provides an economic benefit to the whole country, so public funds should be used to support schools.
C) Although many people never use a hospital, we should still use public funds to provide them, because many people cannot afford private healthcare, and thus we need a publically available health service for those people.
D) There is no evidence that the fire service provides any benefit to the majority of the public, who will never experience a house fire in their lifetime. Thus, the fire service should not be publically funded via taxation.
E) The Police service is a vital service for the country so should be publically funded regardless of how few people benefit from its presence.

Question 28:

SpicNSpan Inc is a cleaning company offering a range of cleaning services across the UK. The board has recently acquired a new chairman, who has called a meeting of the board to assess how the company can move forwards, expanding its services and increasing its market share. One of the things the new chairman is looking at is the types of services the company provides. He argues that their "All inclusive" service, where customers pay a fixed amount to clean a house throughout as a one-off event, are more popular than their "Hourly" services, where customers pay for a cleaner to carry out a certain number of hours each week. The new chairman argues that they should therefore focus on the "All inclusive services", rather than the "Hourly" services, in order to increase profits.

Which of the following best illustrates a flaw in the Chairman's argument?

A) The company offers other services which may bring in even more profit than All Inclusive Services
B) The fact that All inclusive services are more popular than Hourly services does not mean that they are more profitable. Hourly services may be more profitable.
C) He has assumed that hourly services are more popular than All inclusive services
D) He has assumed that all inclusive services are more popular than hourly services
E) The rest of the board may have other strategies to increase profits, which are better than the new Chairman's.

Question 29:

The effects of fossil fuels such as Oil, Coal and Natural gas on the environment are plain and clear for everybody to see. The long-term use of such non-renewable fuels to produce power has led to devastating climate change, and will continue to cause damage as long as it continues. With this in mind, the European Commission has devised a set of targets to promote energy production by different types of fuels. However, there is a glaring problem with these targets. Shockingly, the Commission has targeted a "150% increase in the amount of energy produced by Nuclear Power by 2025". This is an outrageous misjudgement, because Nuclear Power is a non-renewable fuel, just like Oil, Coal and Natural gas. If we wish to protect the environment and halt climate change, we need to switch to *renewable* fuels, which are proven not to cause damage to the environment, NOT non-renewables such as Nuclear.

Which of the following best illustrates a flaw in this passage?

A) It has assumed that all non-renewable power sources cause environmental damage.
B) It has assumed that renewable energy sources do not cause environmental damage.
C) It has assumed that the targets will be met, when in fact there is no guarantee that this will happen.
D) It has neglected to consider other problems with the targets set by the Commission.
E) It has assumed that the climate change caused by burning of oil, coal and natural gas cannot be offset or prevented by other strategies.

Question 30:

Despite the overwhelming evidence which certifies that vaccines are a miracle of modern medicine, and are responsible for saving a great number of lives, there remains a stubborn section of society that refuses to take vaccinations against important diseases, insisting that they are unsafe and ineffective. This group maintain this view in spite of extremely strong evidence that vaccines are safe, and against advice given by doctors. This group is particularly strong in the USA, where they pose a very real concern. Over the last 5 years, the proportion of the population that is unvaccinated has been rising by 1 each year, such that now a staggering 6% of Americans have not received any vaccinations.

Experts have advised that due to the way diseases are spread, if less than 90% of the population at any given time is unvaccinated, then it is almost certain that we will see an outbreak of Measles, a highly contagious and damaging disease. Thus, we expect that there will likely be an outbreak of measles in the next 5 years in the USA, and we should take steps to prepare for this.

Which of the following, if true, would most *strengthen* this argument?

A) New and powerful evidence of the safety of vaccinations is due to be released to the public next year.
B) Measles is a highly damaging disease, which frequently causes death or severe permanent injury in those affected.
C) Throughout the last half-century, the number of people who are not vaccinated has risen and fallen continuously. Usually, the increases in non-vaccinated individuals occur over a 6-year period, after which time vaccination becomes more popular, and this number falls.
D) The number of doctors advising against vaccination has been rising for the last 10 years, and shows no signs of decreasing.
E) The rise in unvaccinated individuals has been increasing steadily for 5 years. The only time such a rate of increase has occurred in history was during the 1950s/1960s. In this case, a similar rate of increase in non-vaccinated individuals was maintained for a staggering 13 years.

Question 31:

PREDICTED

	A	B	C	D	E	U
A	7	4	2	1	0	0
B	3	8	2	2	1	0
C	2	4	5	7	3	1
D	2	2	2	6	5	0
E	1	2	2	1	7	2
U	1	1	0	3	5	6

(ACTUAL, along the left side)

The table above shows the actual and predicted AS grades for 100 AS mathematics students at Greentown Sixth Form. Each student is only predicted one grade. What percentage of students had their grades correctly predicted?

A) 14%   B) 16%   C) 39%   D) 61%   E) 78%

Question 32:

In one year, Mike lowers his workers' wages by x%. The next year, he lowers their wages by x%. The year after this, he raises the wages by x%. In the final year, he raises their wages by x%. In all these stages, x is a constant positive number.

Compared to the workers' original wages before any raising or lowering, what are their new wages?

A) The same as the original wages
B) Lower than the original wages
C) Higher than the original wages
D) Can't tell from the provided information even if we know what x was
E) Can't tell from the provided information but would be able to tell if we knew what x was.

END OF SECTION

Section 2

Question 1:
Why do cells undergo mitosis?

1. Asexual Reproduction
2. Sexual Reproduction

3. Growth of the human embryo
4. Replacement of dead cells

A) 1 only
B) 2 only
C) 3 only

D) 4 only
E) 2 and 3
F) 1, 2, and 3

G) 1, 3, and 4
H) 2, 3, and 4

Question 2:
A ball of radius 2 m and density 3 kg/m^3 is released from the top of a frictionless ramp of height 20m and rolls down. What is its speed at the bottom? Take $\pi = 3$ and $g = 10\text{m}^{-2}$.

A) 1 ms^{-1}
B) 4 ms^{-1}

C) 7 ms^{-1}
D) 9 ms^{-1}

E) 14 ms^{-1}
F) 20 ms^{-1}

Question 3:
Which of the following statements regarding transition metals is correct?

A) Transition metals usually form covalent bonds.
B) Transition metals cannot be used as catalysts as they are too reactive.
C) Transition metals form ions that have multiple colours.
D) Transition metals are poor conductors of electricity.
E) Transition metals are frequently referred to as f-block elements.

Question 4:
Which of the following statements is true regarding waves?

A) Waves can transfer mass in the direction of propagation.
B) All waves have the same energy.
C) All light waves have the same energy.
D) Waves can interfere with each other.
E) None of the above.

The following information applies to questions 5 - 6:

Professor Huang accidentally touches a hot pan and her hand moves away in a reflex action. The diagram below shows a schematic of the reflex arc involved.

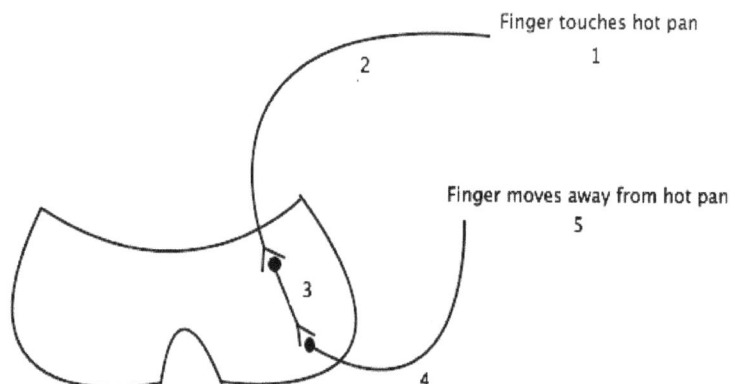

Question 5:
Which option correctly identifies the labels in the pathway?

	Muscle	Sensory Neurone	Receptor	Motor Neurone
A)	1	2	3	4
B)	2	3	1	5
C)	5	2	1	4
D)	1	4	5	2
E)	3	4	5	2
F)	4	2	1	3

Question 6:
Which one of the following statements is correct?

1. Information passes between 1 and 2 chemically.
2. Information passes between 2 and 3 electrically.
3. Information passes between 3 and 4 chemically.

A) 1 only
B) 2 only
C) 3 only
D) 1 and 2
E) 2 and 3
F) 1 and 3
G) All of the above
H) None of the above

Question 7:
Which of the following correctly describes the product of the reaction between hydrochloric acid and but-2-ene?

A) $CH_3-CH_2-C(Cl)H-CH_3$
B) $CH_3-C(Cl)-CH_2-CH_3$
C) $C(Cl)H_2-CH_2-CH_2-CH_3$
D) $CH_3-CH_2-CH_2-C(Cl)H_2$
E) None of the above.

Question 8:

Rearrange $\frac{(7x+10)}{(9x+5)} = 3z^2 + 2$, to make x the subject.

A.

B.

C.

D.

E.

F. $x = \frac{15z^2}{7 + 3(3z^2+2)}$

Question 9:

The electrolysis of brine can be represented by the following equation: $2\,NaCl + 2\,X = 2\,Y + Z + Cl_2$
What are the correct formulae for X, Y and Z?

	X	Y	Z
A)	H_2O	H_2	O_2
B)	H_2O	NaOH	O_2
C)	H_2O	NaOH	H_2
D)	H_2	H_2O	O_2
E)	H_2	NaOH	O_2
F)	H_2	NaOH	H_2
G)	NaOH	H_2O	H_2
H)	NaOH	H_2O	O_2

Question 10:

Element $^{188}_{90}X$ decays into two equal daughter nuclei after a single alpha decay and the release of gamma radiation. What is the daughter element?

A) $^{91}_{45}D$

B) $^{92}_{44}D$

C) $^{184}_{88}D$

D) $^{186}_{90}D$

E) $^{186}_{45}D$

Question 11:

An unknown element has two isotopes: ^{76}X and ^{78}X. $A_r = 76.5$. Which of the statements below are true of X?

1. ^{76}X is three times as abundant as ^{78}X.
2. ^{78}X is three times as abundant as ^{76}X.
3. ^{76}X is more stable than ^{78}X.

A) 1 only

B) 2 only

C) 3 only

D) 1 and 3

E) 2 and 3

F) None of the above.

Question 12:

For the following reaction, which of the statements below is true?

$$6CO_2\,{(g)} + 6H_2O \rightarrow C_6H_{12}O_6 + 6O_2\,{(g)}$$

A) Increasing the concentration of the products will increase the reaction rate.

B) Whether this reaction will proceed at room temperature is independent of the entropy.

C) The reaction rate can be monitored by measuring the volume of gas released.

D) This reaction represents aerobic respiration.

E) This reaction represents anaerobic respiration.

Question 13:
Which of the following are true about the formation of polymers?

1.   They are formed from saturated molecules.
2.   Water is released when polymers form.
3.   Polymers only form linear molecules.

A)   Only 1   D)   1 and 2   G)   All of the above.
B)   Only 2   E)   1 and 3   H)   None of the above.
C)   Only 3   F)   2 and 3

Question 14:
The diagram below shows a series of identical sports fields:

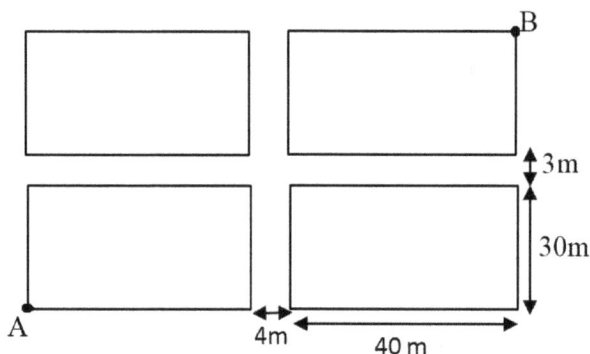

Calculate the shortest distance between points A and B.

A) 100 m   C) 146 m   E) 154 m
B) 105 m   D) 148 m   F) None of the above.

Question 15:
Calculate $\dfrac{1.25 \times 10^{10} + 1.25 \times 10^{9}}{2.5 \times 10^{8}}$

A) 0   D) 110   G)
B) 1   E)
C) 55   F)

The following information applies to questions 16 - 17:

Duchenne muscular dystrophy (DMD) is inherited in an X-linked recessive pattern [transmitted on the X chromosome and requires the absence of normal X chromosomes to result in disease]. A man with DMD has two boys with a woman carrier.

Question 16:
What is the probability that both boys have DMD?

A) 100%   B) 75%   C) 50%   D) 25%   E) 12.5%   F) 0%

Question 17:
If the same couple had two more children, what is the probability that they are both girls with DMD?

A) 100%   B) 75%   C) 50%   D) 25%   E) 12.5%   F) 0%

Question 18:

Which row of the table is correct regarding the cell shown below?

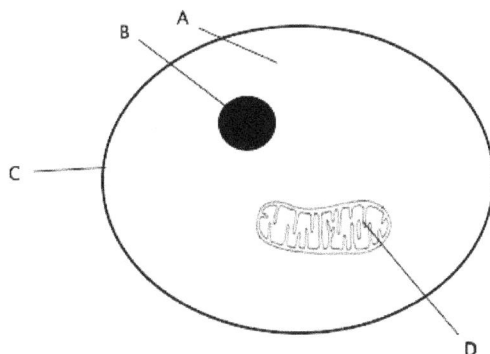

	Most Chemical Reactions occur here	**Involved in Energy Release**	**Cell Type**
A)	A	B	Animal
B)	A	B	Bacterial
C)	A	D	Animal
D)	B	D	Bacterial
E)	B	B	Animal
F)	B	A	Bacterial
G)	D	D	Animal
H)	D	B	Bacterial

Question 19:

Solve $y = 2x - 1$ and $y = x^2 - 1$ for x and y.

A) (0, -1) and (2, 3)   C) (1, 4) and (3, 2)   E) (3, -1) and (3, 1)

B) (1, -1) and (2, 2)   D) (2, -3) and (4, 5)   F) (4, -2) and (-2, 4)

Question 20:

Tim stands at the waterfront and holds a 30 cm ruler horizontally at eye level one metre in front of him. It lines up so it appears to be exactly the same length as a cruise ship 1 km out to sea. How long is the cruise ship?

A) 299.7 m   B) 300.0 m   C) 333.3 m   D) 29,970 m   E) 30,000 m

Question 21:

Which of the following Energy-Temperature graphs best represents the melting of ice to water?

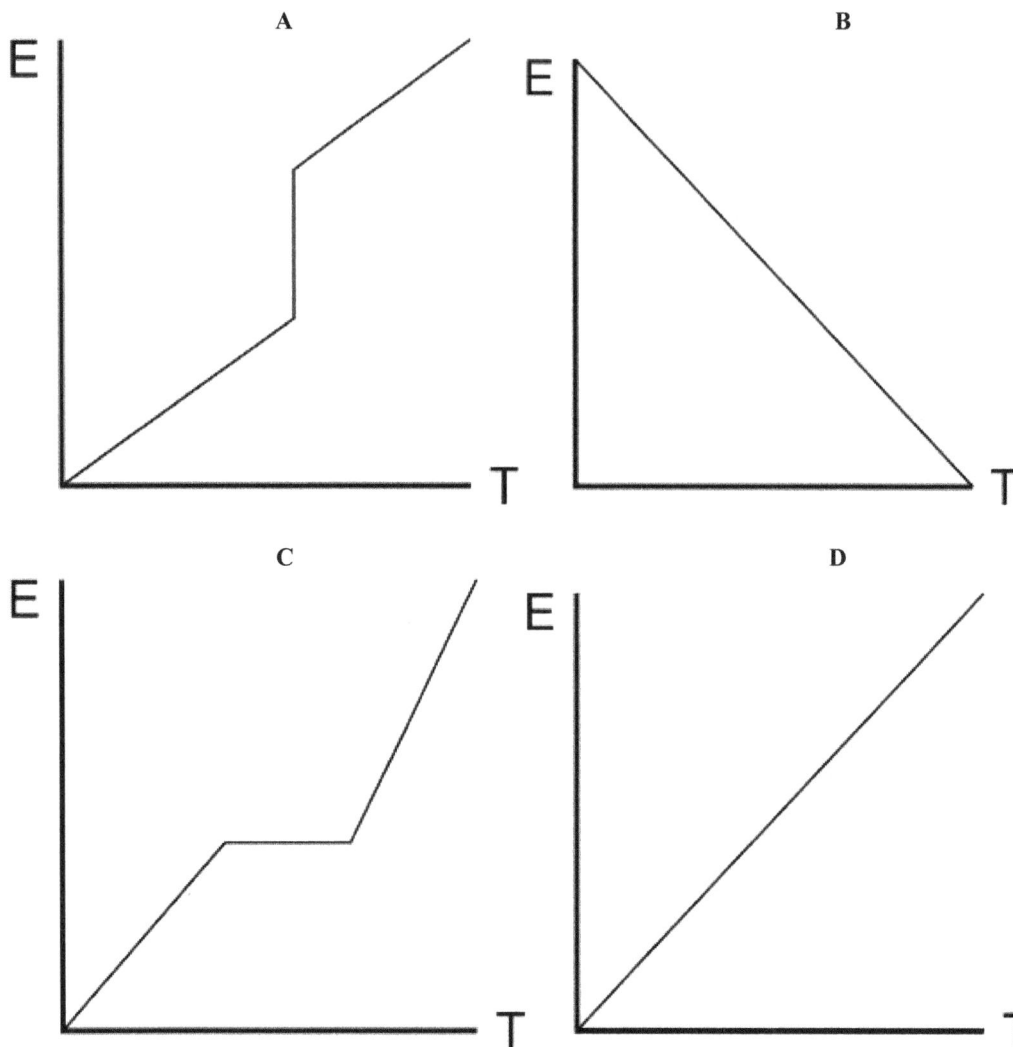

Question 22:

Which of the following statements about white blood cells is correct?

1. They act by engulfing pathogens such as bacteria.
2. They are able to kill pathogens.
3. They transport carbon dioxide away from dying cells.

A)	Only 1	C)	Only 3	E)	2 and 3	G)	All
B)	Only 2	D)	1 and 2	F)	1 and 3	H)	None

Question 23:

Which of the following statements is true regarding the Doppler Effect?

A)   The Doppler Effect applies only to sounds.
B)   The Doppler Effect makes ambulances appear to have a higher frequency when driving towards you.
C)   The Doppler Effect makes ambulances sound higher-pitched when driving away from you.
D)   The Doppler Effect means you never hear the real siren sound as an ambulance drives past.

Question 24:

A 1.2 V battery is rated at 2500 mA hours and is used to power a 30 W light. How many batteries will it take to power the light for 1 hour?

A)   1   B)   6   C)   10   D)   60   E)   100

Question 25:

When electricity flows through a metal, which of the following are true?

1.   Ions move through the metal to create a current.
2.   The lattice in the metal is broken.
3.   Only electrons which were already free of their atoms will flow.

A)   1 only   C)   3 only   E)   1 and 3
B)   2 only   D)   1 and 2   F)   2 and 3

Question 26:

A man cycles along a road at the rate shown in the graph below.

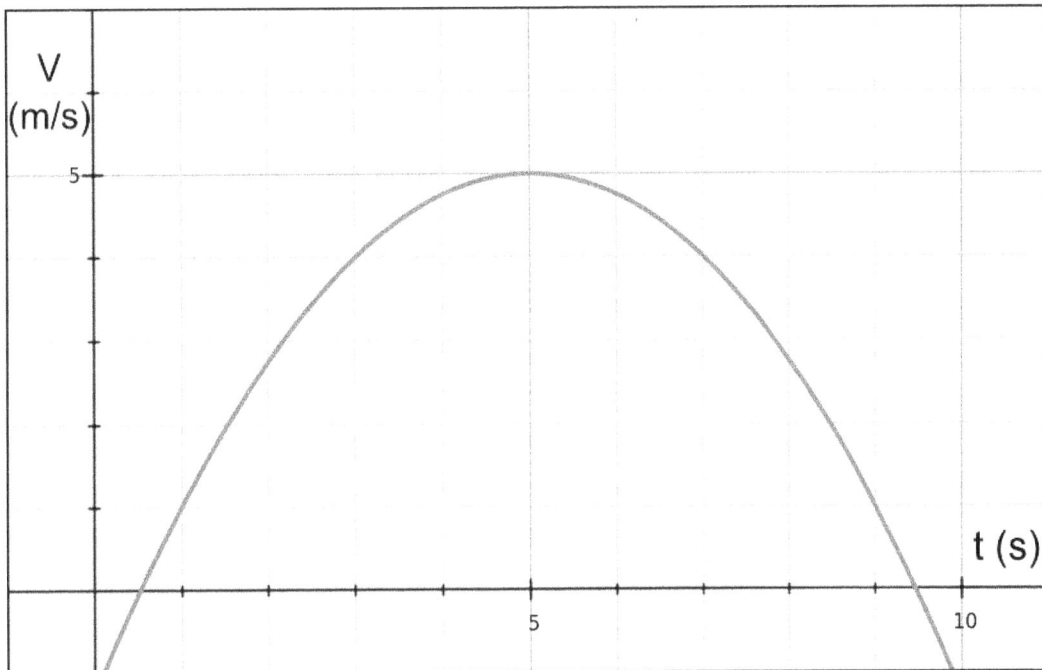

Calculate his displacement at t = 10 seconds.

A)   5 m   C)   25 m   E)   35 m
B)   10 m   D)   30 m   F)   40m

Question 27:

Bob is twice as old as Kerry, and Kerry is three times as old as Bob's son. Their ages combined make 50 years. How old was Bob when his son was born?

A)   15   B)   20   C)   25   D)   30   E)   35

END OF SECTION

Section 3

1) *'A doctor should never disclose medical information about his patients'*

What does this statement mean? Argue to the contrary using examples to strengthen your response. To what extent do you agree with this statement?

2) *'Science is nothing more than just a thought process'*

Explain what this statement means. Argue to the contrary, that science is much more than just a thought process. To what extent, if any, do you agree with the statement?

3) *'With an ageing population, it's necessary to increase the individual's contribution to the healthcare system in order to maintain standards.'*

Explain what this statement means. Argue to the contrary. To what extent do you agree with the statement?

4) *'Assisted suicide allows those suffering from incurable diseases to die with dignity and without unnecessary pain.'*

Explain what this statement means. Argue the contrary. To what extent do you agree with the statement?

END OF PAPER

MOCK PAPER G

Section 1

Question 1:

Irish Folk Band, the Willow, have recently signed a contract with a new manager, and are organising a new musical tour. They and their manager are discussing which country would be best to organise their tour in. The lead singer of the willow would like to organise a tour in Germany, which has a rich history of folk music. However, the new manager finds that ticket sales for folk music concerts in Germany have been steadily declining for several years, whilst France has recently seen a significant increase in ticket sales for folk music concerts. The manager says that this means the group's ticket sales would be higher if they organise a tour in France, than if they organise one in Germany.

Which of the following is an assumption that the manager has made?

A) The band should prioritise profits and organise a tour in the most profitable country possible.
B) The band should not embark upon a new tour and should instead focus on record sales.
C) The decrease of ticket sales in Germany and the increase in France means that the band will sell fewer tickets in Germany than in France.
D) There will not be other countries which are even more profitable than France to organise the tour in.
E) Folk music is popular in France.

Question 2:

Wendy is sending 50 invitations to her housewarming party by first class post. Every envelope contains an invitation weighing 70g, and some who are going to family and friends who live further away also contain a sheet of directions, which weigh 25g. The table below gives the prices of sending letters of certain weights by first or second class post.

If the total cost of sending the invitations is £33, how many of the invitations contain the extra information?

	First Class	Second Class
Less than 50g	£0.50	£0.30
Less than 75g	£0.60	£0.40
Less than 100g	£0.70	£0.50
Less than 125g	£0.80	£0.60
Less than 150g	£0.90	£0.70

A) 15   B) 20   C) 25   D) 30   E) 35

Question 3:

Grace and Rose have both been attending an afterschool gymnastics class, which finishes at 5pm. After the class has finished, Grace and Rose cool down and change out of their gym clothes before heading home. Both girls depart at 5:15pm. Grace and Rose both live a 1.5 mile walk away from the local gymnasium. Therefore, they will definitely arrive home at the same time.

Which of the following is **NOT** an assumption made in this argument?

A) Both girls will walk at the same speed.
B) Both girls departed at the same time.
C) The gymnastics class is being held at the local gymnasium.
D) Grace will not get lost on the way home.
E) Both girls are walking home.

Question 4:

John is a train enthusiast, who has been studying the directions in which trains travel after departing from various London Stations. He finds that Trains departing from King's Cross station in London head North on the East Coast Mainline, and travel to Edinburgh. Trains departing from Waterloo Station head West on the Southwest Mainline and travel to Plymouth. Trains departing from Victoria Station head South and travel to Kent.

John surmises that presently, in order to travel on a train from London to Edinburgh, he must get on at King's Cross Station.

Which of the following is an assumption that John has made?

A) The East Coast mainline has the fastest trains.

B) It would not be quicker to take a train from Waterloo to Southampton Airport, then travel to Edinburgh on an Aeroplane.

C) Rail lines will not be built that will allow trains to travel from Waterloo Station or Victoria Station to Edinburgh.

D) King's Cross trains do not have any other destinations other than Edinburgh.

E) There are no other train stations in London from which trains may travel to Edinburgh.

Question 5:

Summer and Shaniqua are playing a game of "noughts and crosses". Each player is assigned either "noughts" (O) or "crosses" (X) and they take it in turns to choose an empty box of the 3x3 grid to put their symbol in. The winner is the first person to get a line of 3 of their symbol in any direction in the grid (vertically, horizontally or diagonally). Summer starts the game. The current position is shown below:

X	X	
	O	

Assuming Shaniqua now plays her symbol in the square which will stop Summer being able to win the game straight away, Summer should play in either of which 2 boxes to ensure she is able to win the game on the next turn no matter what Shaniqua does?

1	2	3
		4
6		5

A) 1 and 3   B) 1 and 5   C) 1 and 6   D) 2 and 4   E) 3 and 5

Question 6:

Tanks and armoured vehicles were a hugely influential factor in all battles in World War 2. German tanks were highly superior to the tanks used by France, and this was an essential reason why Germany was able to defeat France in 1940. However, Germany was later defeated in World War 2 by the Soviet Union. Germany lost a number of key battles such as the Battle of Stalingrad and the Battle of Kursk. These victories were essential for the eventual victory of the Soviet Union over Germany. Therefore, the Soviet Union's tanks in the battles of Stalingrad and Kursk must have been superior to those of Germany.

Which of the following is an assumption made in this argument?

A) Tanks were hugely influential in the Battle of Stalingrad.

B) The Battles of Stalingrad and Kursk were essential for the Soviet Union's victory over Germany.

C) The reasons why the Soviet Union defeated Germany in battle were the same as the reasons why Germany defeated France in battle.

D) German tanks being superior to those used by France was an essential reason why Germany was able to defeat France.

E) If the Soviet Union's tanks were superior to Germany's tanks, the Soviet Union's armoured vehicles must also have been superior to Germany's armoured vehicles.

Question 7:

In the Battle of Waterloo, in 1815, French Emperor Napoleon Bonaparte's army was defeated by a British army commanded by British General Arthur Wellesley, Duke of Wellington. Essential to The British army's victory was the arrival of a group of Prussian reinforcements led by Field Marshal Von Blucher, which joined up with The British army and allowed them to overwhelm Bonaparte's left flank. Bonaparte had been aware of the threat posed by Von Blucher's Prussians, and had detached a force of French soldiers several days earlier under the command of Field Marshal Grouchy, with orders to engage the Prussians led by Von Blucher, and prevent them joining up with The British Army.

However, whilst dining at a local inn, Grouchy mistook the sounds of gunfire for thunder, and believed that the battle had been cancelled. He therefore disobeyed his orders and did not engage the Prussians commanded by Von Blucher. Therefore, if Field Marshal Grouchy had not made this mistake and had engaged the Prussian force as commanded, The British would not have won the Battle of waterloo.

Which is the best statement of a flaw in this argument?

A) It implies Field Marshal Grouchy was an incompetent commander, when in fact he was a highly respected general of the day.

B) It assumes that had Grouchy engaged the Prussian force, he would have been able to successfully prevent them joining up with the British army.

C) It assumes that the British army would not have been victorious without the arrival of the Prussian reinforcements.

D) It ignores the other mistakes made by Napoleon which contributed to the British army being victorious in the Battle of Waterloo.

E) It implies that thunder and gunshot sounds are frequently mistaken by generals.

Question 8:

A cruise ship is sailing from Southampton to Barcelona, making several stops along the way at Calais and Bordeux, in France, Bilbao in Spain, and Porto in Portugal. At each stop, the ship must wait in a queue to be assigned a Dock at which it can pull in, refuel and resupply. The busier the port, the longer the ship will have to queue to be assigned a Dock. The Captain of the ship is planning the journey, and knows he must work out which ports will have the longest queues.

The Captain made the same journey last year, and found out that Bilbao was the busiest port in Europe during the course of the journey. He also knows that Bordeux is the busiest port in France, and that Porto is the busiest port in Portugal. Whilst he is planning the journey, he discovers that Calais is busier than Porto. The Captain concludes that he must plan for Bilbao to have the longest queue in the journey, Bordeux to have the second longest queue, Calais to have the third longest queue, and Porto to have the fourth longest queue.

Which of the following best illustrates a flaw in the Captain's Reasoning?

A) Porto is less busy than Calais, but may be busier than Bordeux.
B) The rankings may have changed and Bilbao may no longer be the busiest port in Europe.
C) Just because a port is busier does not necessarily mean it will have the longest queues.
D) The ship may not have time to make all the stops.
E) The captain has forgotten to consider how many passengers will embark and disembark at each stop.

Question 9:

A packaging company wishes to make cardboard boxes by taking a flat 1.2 m by 1.2 m square piece of cardboard, cutting square sections out of each corner as shown by the picture below and folding up the sections remaining on each side to make a box. The company experiments with different size boxes by cutting differently sized squares from the corners each time. It makes a box with 10 cm by 10 cm squares cut out of each corner, a box with 20 cm by 20 cm squares cut out of each corner and so on up to one with 50 cm by 50 cm squares cut out of each corner.

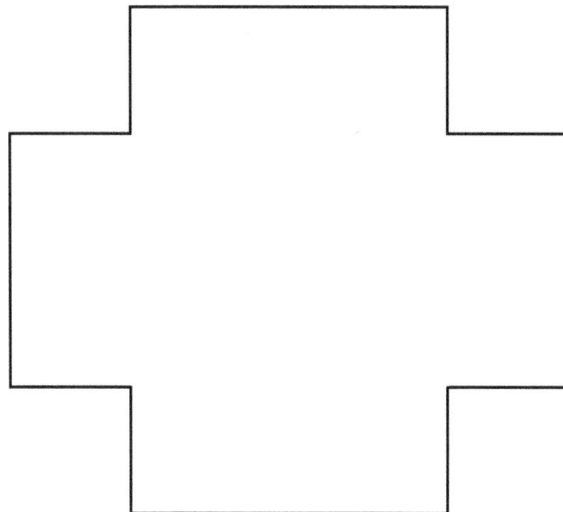

Which side length cut out would result in a box with the largest volume?

A) 10 cm   B) 20 cm   C) 30 cm   D) 40 cm   E) 50 cm

Question 10:

The aeroplane was a marvel of modern engineering when it was first developed in the early 20th Century, and was testament to human ingenuity. Throughout the 20th Century, the aeroplane allowed humans to travel more freely and widely than ever before, and allowed people to see and appreciate the stunning natural beauty the world has to offer. However, Aeroplanes also produce lots of pollution, such as Carbon Dioxide and Sulphur Oxide. High levels of Carbon Dioxide in the atmosphere are currently causing global warming, which is destroying or damaging many natural environments throughout the world.

Therefore it is clear that the aeroplane, which once offered such opportunity to appreciate the world's natural beauty, has been largely responsible for damage to various natural environments throughout the world. We must now seek to curb air traffic in order to save the world's remaining natural environments.

Which of the following is the best statement of a flaw in this argument?

A) It assumes that aeroplanes are a major reason for the high levels of Carbon Dioxide in the atmosphere which are currently causing global warming.
B) It assumes that aeroplanes offer greater opportunity to appreciate the world's natural environments.
C) It assumes that high levels of Carbon Dioxide are responsible for global warming.
D) It does not consider the effects of Sulphur Dioxide pollution released by aeroplanes.
E) It implies that we should take action to prevent damage to the world's natural environments.

Question 12:

Professors from the department of Pathology at Oxford University are conducting research into possible new treatments for malaria, which is caused by a microbe known as Plasmodium. Research from Sierra Leone, a third world country with a high rate of malaria, has found that liver cells in malaria patients are reactive to the antibody Tarpulin. Plasmodium is known to infect liver cells, and thus liver cells would react to Tarpulin if Plasmodium itself was reactive to Tarpulin. Thus, the professors at Oxford begin to research how Tarpulin can be used to target Plasmodium and treat malaria.

However, this research will not be successful, because liver cells would also react to Tarpulin if the wrong solution is used whilst conducting the experiments. Since malaria is not prevalent in Oxford, the professors must rely on the data from Sierra Leone. If the experiments in Sierra Leone used the wrong solutions, then the liver cells would react to Tarpulin even if Plasmodium does not react to Tarpulin.

Which of the following best illustrates a flaw in this argument?

A) From the fact that Plasmodium infects liver cells, it cannot be inferred that infected liver cells would react to Tarpulin if Plasmodium does.
B) From the fact that the research was carried out in Sierra Leone, it cannot be inferred that the wrong solutions were used.
C) From the fact that the wrong solutions are used, it cannot be inferred that the liver cells would react to Tarpulin.
D) From the fact that Plasmodium is reactive to Tarpulin it cannot be assumed that Tarpulin can be used to combat Plasmodium.
E) From the fact that Liver cells react to Tarpulin, it cannot be inferred that Plasmodium is reactive to Tarpulin.

Question 12:

Ancient Egypt was one of the world's most powerful nations for several thousand years, and wondrous structures such as the Sphinxes and the Great Pyramids serve as a permanent reminder of its stature. Many other powerful nations throughout the ages have also built magnificent structures, such as the Colosseum built by the Romans, the Hanging Gardens of Babylon built by the Persians and the Great Wall of China built by the Chinese. As well as building magnificent structures, Rome, Persia and China had one other thing in common, namely a very strong military. Thus, history clearly shows us that in ancient times, for a nation to be a powerful nation, it must have had a very strong military. In addition to building great structures such as the pyramids, Ancient Egypt must have also possessed a very strong military.

Which of the following best illustrates the main conclusion of this argument?

A) In order to be a powerful nation, a nation must build magnificent structures.
B) In Ancient times a very strong military was required to be a powerful nation.
C) Ancient Egypt built magnificent structures; therefore it must have been a powerful nation.
D) Rome, Persia and China were all powerful nations.
E) Ancient Egypt was a powerful nation; therefore it must have had a very strong military.

Question 13:

Global warming is widely presented in modern society as a cause for significant concern. One particular area often thought to be at risk is the Ice caps of the North and South Poles, which are often presented to be at risk of melting due to increased temperature. Environmentalist groups often campaign for energy consumption to be reduced, thus reducing CO_2 emissions, the leading cause of global warming. However, recent research shows that the North and South Poles are actually becoming cooler, not warmer, thanks to mysterious and unexplained weather patterns. Clearly, high energy consumption is not contributing to damage to the Polar Ice caps.

Which of the following statements can be reliably inferred from this argument?

A) There is no point in reducing energy consumption for environmental reasons.
B) Reducing energy consumption will not reduce CO_2 emissions.
C) We should trust the recent research stating that the North and South poles are becoming cooler.
D) Reducing energy consumption will not contribute to saving the polar ice caps.
E) We should not be concerned about damage to the Polar Ice caps.

Question 14:

In 1957 the drug Thalidomide was released, and used to relieve nausea and morning sickness during pregnancy. The pharmaceutical company which released Thalidomide had carried out extensive testing of the drug, and had carried out more tests than was required for new drugs in the 1950s. No adverse affects were reported, and the drug was thought to be safe and effective. However, after it was released, Thalidomide was found to be responsible for severe deformities in thousands of babies whose mothers had taken the drug whilst pregnant with them. When further research was carried out, it was found that the molecules in Thalidomide could adopt 2 molecular structures, known as isomers. One of these isomers was perfectly safe, but the other caused significant biological problems in pregnant women and had been responsible for the deformities in the babies. The company producing Thalidomide had not been aware of this 2nd isomer when developing the drug.

Which of the following is a conclusion that can be drawn from this passage?

A) The company producing Thalidomide had acted irresponsibly by not carrying out the required level of testing for the drug.
B) No isomers of Thalidomide are safe.
C) The drug testing requirements in 1950s were not sufficient to identify all possible isomers of a given drug.
D) Thalidomide was not effective at relieving nausea and morning sickness.
E) The dangerous isomer of Thalidomide was not effective at relieving nausea and morning sickness.

Question 15:

A teacher is trying to arrange the 5 students in her class into a seating plan. Her classroom contains 2 tables, arranged one behind the other, which each sit 3 people. Ashley must sit on the front row on the left hand side nearest the board because she has poor eyesight. Bella and Caitlin must not be sat in the same row as each other because they talk and disrupt the class. Danielle needs to be sat next to an empty seat as she sometimes has help from a teaching assistant. Emily should be sat on the end of a row because she has poor mobility and it is hard for her to get into a middle seat.

Who is sitting in the front right seat?

A) Empty   B) Bella   C) Caitlin   D) Danielle   E) Emily

Question 16:

The release of CO_2 from consumption of fossil fuels is the main reason behind global warming, which is causing significant damage to many natural environments throughout the world. One significant source of CO_2 emissions is cars, which release CO_2 as they use up petrol. In order to tackle this problem, many car companies have begun to design cars with engines that do not use as much petrol. However, engines which use less petrol are not as powerful, and less powerful cars are not attractive to the public. If a car company produces cars which are not attractive to the public, they will not be profitable.

Which of the following best illustrates the main conclusion of this argument?

A) Car companies which produce cars that use less petrol will not be profitable.
B) The public prefer more powerful cars.
C) Car companies should prioritise profits over helping the environment.
D) Car companies should seek to produce engines that use less petrol but are still just as powerful.
E) The public are not interested in helping the environment.

Question 17:

Penicillin is one of the major success stories of modern medicine. Since its discovery in 1928, it has grown to become a crucial foundation of medicine, saving countless lives and introducing the age of antibiotics. Alexander Fleming is today given most of the credit for introducing and developing antibiotics, but in fact Fleming played a relatively minor role. Fleming initially discovered Penicillin, but was unable to demonstrate its clinical effectiveness, or discern ways of reliably and consistently producing it. 2 other scientists called Howard Florey and Ernst Chain were actually responsible for developing Penicillin to the point where it could be reliably produced and used in medicine, to treat infections in patients. Clearly, the credit for the wonders worked by Penicillin should not go to Fleming, but to Florey and Chain.

Which of the following best illustrates the main conclusion of this argument?

A) Fleming was unable to develop penicillin to the point of being a viable medical treatment.
B) The credit for Penicillin's effects on medicine should go to Ernst Chain and Howard Florey, not to Alexander Fleming.
C) Without Chain and Florey, Penicillin would not have been developed into a viable treatment.
D) Alexander Fleming only played a small role in the process of Penicillin becoming a feature of modern medicine.
E) Alexander Fleming is not given enough credit for his role in the development of penicillin.

Question 18:

I write my 4 digit pin number down in a coded format, by multiplying the first and second number together, dividing by the third number than subtracting the fourth number. If my code is 3, which of these could my pin number be?

A) 3461   B) 9864   C) 5423   D) 7848   E) 6849

Question 19:

Worcestershire Aquatic Centre is a business seeking to recruit a new dolphin trainer. They interview several candidates, and find that there are 2 candidates which are clearly more suitable than the others. They give both of these candidates a 2nd interview, with further questions about their experience and qualifications.

They discern that Candidate 1 has a proven capability to perform well to crowds, which is likely to bring in more profit to the Aquatic Centre as more people will come and watch a more entertaining dolphin show. However, unlike Candidate 1, Candidate 2 has experience at handling dolphins, and a proven ability to maximise their welfare standards. The manager of the aquatic centre tells the recruiting officer to prioritise profits, and therefore to hire Candidate 1.

Which of the following statements, if true, would most *weaken* the manager's argument?

A) Market research conducted by an external organisation showed that 60% of members of the public would be more likely to attend a dolphin show presented by a charismatic host.

B) Candidate 1's performance experience was not in the aquatic industry.

C) Other aquatic centres with poor welfare standards have been subject to negative media attention and subsequent boycotts.

D) A local charity-run aquatic centre have decided to prioritise donkey welfare and their manager recommends such a strategy.

E) A well-respected business analyst predicts that profit will rise under Candidate 2.

Question 20:

Rental yield for buy to let properties is calculated by dividing the potential rent per year paid for a house by the amount it cost to buy the house and get it in a rentable condition. Tina is considering 5 houses as possible buy to let investments. House A is in good condition and could be rented as it is for £700 a month, and costs £168,000 to buy. House B is also in good condition but is a student house so Tina would need to buy furniture for it. The house would cost £190,000 to buy and £10,000 to furnish, but could be rented for 40 weeks of the year to 4 students at a rent of £125 a week each. House C needs a lot of work doing. It costs £100,000 but would need £44,000 of renovations, and would rent for £600 a month. House D costs £200,000 and would need £40,000 of renovations, and would rent out for £2000 a month. House E costs £80,000 and would need £20,000 of renovations, and could be rented out for £200 a week.

Which house has the highest rental yield?

A) A   B) B   C) C   D) D   E) E

Question 21:

There has recently been a new election in the UK, and the new government is pondering what policy to adopt on the railway system in the UK. The Chancellor argues that the best policy is to have an entirely privatised railway system, which will encourage different train companies to be competitive, and try and attract customers by providing the best service at the lowest price, thus driving down costs and increasing quality for customers. However, the Transport Minister argues that this is a short-sighted policy. She argues that privatised companies will only run services on the most profitable lines, where there are lots of passengers.

Under this system, train companies may not choose to run many services to rural areas. This will lead to rural communities being cut off, with a consequent lack of opportunities for people in these communities. She argues that public funding should be put towards rail services in order to ensure that people in rural communities are adequately served by rail services.

Which of the following, if true, would most strengthen the Transport Minister's argument?

A) The Transport Minister has ultimate power over railway policy, and she can overrule the Chancellor if she sees fit.

B) Many train services to rural communities currently have low passenger numbers, and are unlikely to be profitable.

C) French rail services receive high level of public funding, and users of these services enjoy good quality and low prices.

D) American railway services are privatised with no public funding, and yet rural communities in America are well served by railway services.

E) The Prime Minister agrees with the Transport Minister's line of argument. He sympathises with rural communities and does not believe in a privatised rail system.

Question 22:

Niall can choose whether to join the gym as member or pay per session. Gym membership costs £30 per month but attending classes or gym sessions is free. Pay as you go gym sessions cost £4 and attending classes are £2 each. Niall works out that it will cost him £2 more if he pays per session than it will to buy membership. Which of these is a possible combination of Niall's gym sessions and classes for one month?

A) 5 gym sessions, 4 classes

B) 4 gym sessions, 4 classes

C) 5 gym sessions, 6 classes

D) 4 gym sessions, 6 classes

E) 5 gym sessions, 8 classes

Question 23:

If the mean of 5 numbers is 8, the median is 6 and the mode is 4, what must the two largest numbers in the set of numbers add up to?

A) 13   B) 16   C) 22   D) 26   E) 28

Question 24:

The North York Moors is one of several National Parks in England. The Management team has been awarded a grant from the National Lottery looking for a way to attract more visitors to the Moors. Sam suggests that they invest in enhancing the natural landscapes present in the Moors, thus creating more beauty, and making people more inspired to visit. However, Lucy disagrees, and feels that they should invest in more visitor centres and information points. Lucy's argument that whilst this will be more costly in terms of staffing these centres, the increase in visitor numbers will bring in more income for the Moors, and will counteract this extra cost.

Which of the following, if true, would most *weaken* Lucy's argument?

A) Information Centres in other national parks do not generally generate as much revenue as they cost to staff.
B) National Lottery grants have a history of being badly spent my National Parks such as the North York Moors.
C) There are large numbers of people who are interested in volunteering to help the North York Moors and would be happy to staff visitor centres.
D) Another National Park, the Yorkshire Dales, has recently opened up 5 new visitor centres and seen their profits increase significantly.
E) The North York Moors is currently struggling to attract visitors.

Question 25:

How many different squares (of either 1, 2, 3 or 4 grid squares in side length) can be made using the grid below?

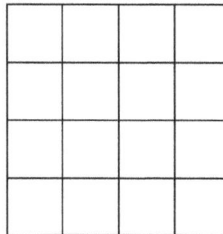

A) 16   B) 20   C) 25   D) 26   E) 30

Question 26:

When I board my train at York at 15:30, the announcer tells me it is 120 minutes to London Kings Cross. Assuming the announcement is accurate to the nearest 10 minutes and that the train is on time, what is the earliest time I might arrive at my destination which is 10 minutes walk from Kings Cross?

A) 17:20   B) 17:25   C) 17:30   D) 17:35   E) 17:40

Question 27:

My sister does 2 loads of washing per week plus an extra one for everyone who is living in the house that week. When her son is away at university, she buys a new carton of washing powder every 6 weeks, but when her son is home she has to buy a new one every 5 weeks. How many people are living in the house when her son is home?

A) 2   B) 3   C) 4   D) 5   E) 6

Question 28:

A train shuttle service runs between the city centre and the airport between 5:30am and 11:30pm on weekdays and 6:00am and midnight on weekends. There are two trains used to operate the service and each journey from the airport to the city centre or vice versa takes 24 minutes. It takes 4 minutes for the train to unload and reload at the airport and 2 minutes for the train to unload and reload at the city centre.

What is the maximum number of single journeys that can be made by the shuttle service in one day?

A) 36   B) 48   C) 60   D) 72   E) 96

Question 29:

Northern Line trains arrive into Waterloo station every 6 minutes, Jubilee Line trains every 2.5 minutes and Bakerloo Line trains every 4 minutes.

If trains from all 3 lines arrived into the station 4 minutes ago, how long will it be before they do so again?

A) 20 minutes   C) 30 minutes   E) 60 minutes

B) 26 minutes   D) 56 minutes

Question 30:

Sam is deciding whether to make her wedding invitations herself or get them professionally made at a cost of £1 each. She decides to work out how much it will cost to make them herself. Each invitation uses 1 sheet of cream card, 4 sheets of red paper and 1 metre of gold ribbon. She will also uses a gold sticker on each invitation and stamp them with a stamper she will buy. The stamper needs a pad of ink which will last for 70 invitations. The table of stationery costs is shown below:

Product	Price
Red paper (pack of 100)	£2
15m roll of gold ribbon	£3
Pack of 30 gold stickers	£1
Stamper	£8
Ink pad	£4
Cream card (pack of 20)	£2

She wants to send 90 invitations and wants to have enough supplies for 4 spares only. How much will she save by making the invitations herself?

A) £15   B) £19   C) £29   D) £31   E) £33

Question 31:

Half of the boys in Mrs Nelson's class have brown eyes and two thirds of the class have brown hair. At least as many boys in the class as girls have brown hair. There are at least as many boys as girls in the class. There are 36 children in the class in total.

What's the minimum number of boys that have both brown hair and brown eyes?

A) 2   B) 3   C) 4   D) 5   E) 6

Question 32:
Mandy is making orange squash for her daughter's birthday party. She wants to have a 300ml glass of squash for each of the 8 children attending and a 400ml glass of squash each for her and for 2 parents who are helping out. She has 600ml of the concentrated squash. What ratio of water:concentrated squash should she use in the dilution to ensure she has the right amount to go around?

A) 7:1   B) 6:1   C) 5:1   D) 4:1   E) 3:1

END OF SECTION

Section 2

Question 1:
Which of the following statements are true?

1. Natural selection always favours organisms that are faster or stronger.
2. Genetic variation leads to different adaptations to the environment.
3. Variation is purely due to genetics.

A) Only 1
B) Only 2
C) Only 3

D) 1 and 2
E) 2 and 3
F) 1 and 3

G) All of the above.
H) None of the above.

Question 2:
Which of the following statements are true about the electrolysis of brine?

1. It describes the reduction of 2 chloride ions to Cl_2.
2. The amount of NaOH produced increases in proportion with the amount of NaCl present in solution, provided there is enough H_2 present to dissolve the NaCl.
3. The redox reaction of the electrolysis of brine results in the production of dissolved NaOH, which is a strong acid.

A) Only 1
B) Only 2
C) Only 3

D) 1 and 2
E) 1 and 3
F) 2 and 3

G) All of the above.
H) None of the above.

The following information applies to questions 3 – 4:

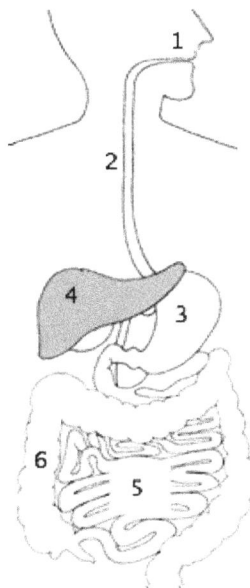

Question 3:
Which of the following numbers indicate where amylase functions?

A) 1 only
B) only

C) 1 and 3
D) 1 and 5

E) 2 and 4
F) 3 and 4

G) 5 and 6

Question 4:

In which of the following does the majority of chemical digestion occur?

A) 1   C) 3   E) 5   G) None of
B) 2   D) 4   F) 6   the above.

Question 5:

Which of the following correctly describes the product of the reaction between propene and hydrofluoric acid (HF)?

A) $C(F)H_3\text{-}CH_2\text{-}CH_3$

B) $CH_3\text{-}C(F)H\text{-}CH_3$

C) $CH_3\text{-}C(F)H_2\text{-}CH_2$

D) $CH_3\text{-}C(F)H_2\text{-}CH_3$

E) None of the above.

Question 6:

Which of the following statements is **FALSE**?

A) A nuclear power plant may have an accident if free neutrons in a fuel rod aren't captured.
B) Humans cannot currently harness the energy from nuclear fusion.
C) Uncontrolled nuclear fission leads to a large explosion.
D) Mass is conserved during nuclear explosions caused by nuclear bombs.
E) Nuclear fusion produces much more energy than nuclear fission.

Question 7:

Which of the following are true about the reaction between alkenes and hydrogen halides?

1. The product formed is fully saturated.
2. The hydrogen halide binds at the alkene's saturated double bond.
3. The hydrogen halide forms ionic bonds with the alkene.

A) Only 1   D) 1 and 2   G) All of the above.
B) Only 2   E) 2 and 3   H) None of the above.
C) Only 3   F) 1 and 3

Question 8:

Rearrange the following to make m the subject.

$$T = 4\pi \sqrt{\frac{(M + 3m)l}{3(M + 2m)g}}$$

A) $m = \frac{16\pi^2 lM - 3gMT^2}{48\pi^2 l - 6gT^2}$

B) $m = \frac{16\pi^2 lM - 3gMT^2}{6gT^2 - 48\pi^2 l}$

C) $m = \frac{3gMT^2 - 16\pi^2 lM}{6gT^2 - 48\pi^2 l}$

D) $m = \frac{4\pi^2 lM - 3gMT^2}{6gT^2 - 16\pi^2 l}$

E) $m = \left(\frac{16\pi^2 lM - 3gMT^2}{6gT^2 - 48\pi^2 l}\right)^2$

Question 9:

Which of the following correctly describes the product of the polymerisation of chloroethene molecules?

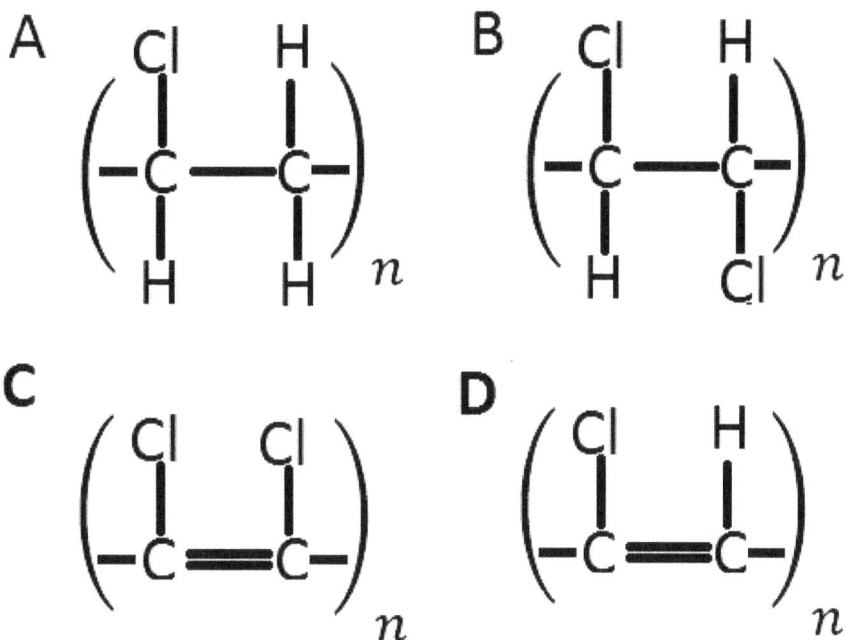

The following information applies to questions 10 – 11:

The diagram below shows the genetic inheritance of colour-blindness, which is inherited in a sex-linked recessive manner [transmitted on the X chromosome and requires the absence of normal X chromosomes to result in disease]. X^B is the normal allele and X^b is the colour-blind allele.

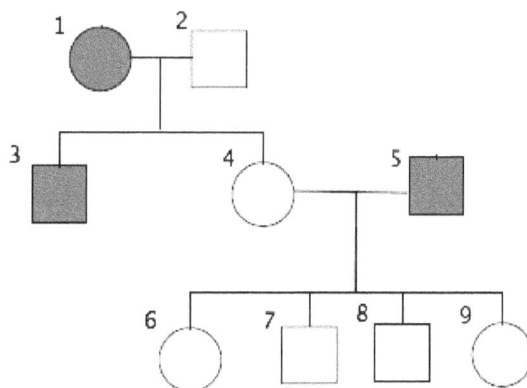

Question 10:

What is the genotype of the individual marked 4?

A) $X^B X^b$ B) $X^B X^B$ C) $X^b X^b$ D) $X^B Y$ E) $X^b Y$

Question 11:

If 8 were to reproduce with a heterozygote female, what is the probability of producing a colour-blind boy?

A) 100%   B) 75%   C) 50%   D) 25%   E) 12.5%   F) 0%

Question 12:

The mean of a set of 11 numbers is 6. Two numbers are removed and the mean is now 5. Which of the following is not a possible combination of removed numbers?

A. 1 and 20
B. 6 and 9

C. 10 and 11
D. 15 and 6

E. 19 and 2

Question 13:

For the following reaction, which of the statements below are true?

$$N_{2(g)} + 3\,H_{2(g)} \rightleftharpoons 2\,NH_{3(g)}$$

1. Increasing pressure will cause the equilibrium to shift to the right.
2. Increasing pressure will form more ammonia gas.
3. Increasing the concentration of N_2 will create more ammonia.

A) 1 only
B) 2 only
A. None of the above.

C) 3 only
D) 1 and 2

E) 2 and 3
F) All of the above.

Question 14:

Find the values of angles b and c.

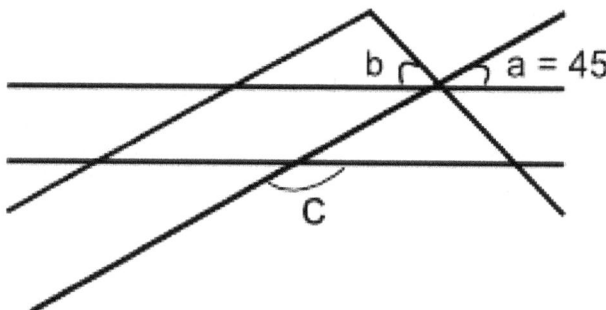

A) 45° and 135°
B) 45° and 130°

C) 50° and 135°
D) 55° and 130°

E) More information needed.

Question 15

When sodium and chlorine react to form salt, which of the following best represents the bonding and electron configurations of the products and reactants?

	Sodium (s)		Chlorine (g)		Salt (s)	
	Intra-element bond	Element electron configuration	Intra-element bond	Element electron configuration	Compound bond	Compound electron configuration
A)	Ionic	2, 8, 1	Covalent	2, 8, 8, 1	Ionic	2, 8, 1 : 2, 8, 8, 1
B)	Metallic	2, 7	Covalent	2, 8, 1	Ionic	2, 8 : 2, 8
C)	Covalent	2, 8, 2	Ionic	2, 8, 8	Covalent	2, 8 : 2, 8, 8
D)	Ionic	2, 7	Ionic	2, 8, 8, 7	Covalent	2, 7 : 2, 8, 8, 7
E)	Metallic	2, 8, 1	Covalent	2, 8, 7	Ionic	2, 8 : 2, 8, 8

Question 16:

Evaluate: $\dfrac{3.4 \times 10^{11} + 3.4 \times 10^{10}}{6.8 \times 10^{12}}$

A)   C)   E)
B)   D)   F)

The following information applies to questions 17 – 18:

In pea plants, colour and stem length are inherited in an autosomal manner. The allele for yellow colour, Y, is dominant to the allele for green colour, y. Furthermore, the allele for tall stem length, T, is dominant to short stem length, t.

When a pea plant of unknown genotype is crossed with a green short-stemmed pea plant, the progeny are 25% yellow + tall-stemmed plants, 25% yellow + short-stemmed plants, 25% green + tall-stemmed plants and 25% green + short-stemmed plants.

Question 17

What is the genotype of the unknown pea plant?

A) Yytt   C) YyTT   E) yyTT
B) YyTt   D) yyTt   F) yytt

Question 18:

Taking both colour and height into account, how many different combinations of genotypes and phenotypes are possible?

A) 6 genotypes and 3 phenotypes   D) 9 genotypes and 4 phenotypes
B) 8 genotypes and 3 phenotypes   E) 9 genotypes and 3 phenotypes
C) 8 genotypes and 4 phenotypes   F) 10 genotypes and 3 phenotypes

Question 19:

Which of the following statements is true regarding electrolysis?

A) Using an AC-current is most effective.
B) Using a DC-current is most effective.
C) An AC-current causes cations to gather at the cathode.
D) A DC-current would plate the anode in copper from a copper sulphate solution.
E) No current is used in electrolysis.

Question 20:

Evaluate the following expression:

$((\frac{6}{8} \times \frac{7}{3}) \div (\frac{7}{5} \times \frac{2}{6})) \times 0.40 \times 15\% \times 5\% \times \pi \times (\sqrt{e^2}) \times 0.20 \times (e\pi)^{-1}$

A)   B)   C)   D)   E)

Question 21:

Which will have a greater current, a circuit with two identical resistors in series or one with the same two resistors in parallel?

A) Series will have greater current than parallel.   C) Same current in both.
B) Parallel will have greater current than series.   D) It depends on the battery.

Question 22:

A 2000 kg car is driving down the road at 36 km per hour. A deer runs out into the road 105 m in front of the car. It takes the driver 0.5 seconds to react to the deer and hit the brakes. The car stops just in time. What is average braking force exerted?

A) 20 N   B) 100 N   C) 200 N   D) 1,000 N   E) 2,000 N

Question 23:

When comparing different isotopes of the same element, which of the following may change?

1. Atomic number
2. Mass number
3. Number of electrons
4. Chemical reactivity

A) 1 only   C) 3 only   E) All of the above

B) 1 and 2 only   D) 2 and 3 only

Question 24:

A man drives along a road as shown in the figure below.

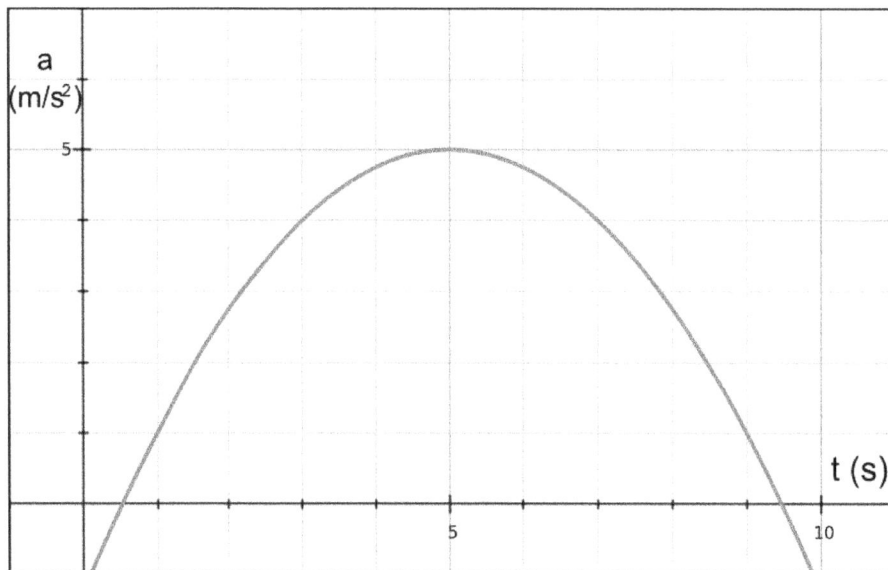

Which of the following statements is true?

A) He drives a total of 30 m.   D) He has an average acceleration of 30 m/s^2.

B) He has an average velocity of 30 m/s.   E) His velocity decreases between 5 and 9 seconds.

C) He has a final velocity of 30 m/s.

Question 25:

A circle has a radius of 3 metres. A line passes through the circle's centre and intersects with a tangent 4 metres from its tangent point. How far is this point of intersection from the centre of the circle?

A) 1 metres   B) 3 metres   C) 5 metres   D) 7 metres   E) 9 metres

Question 26:

Which of the following statements is **FALSE**?

A) Energy cannot be created or destroyed.
B) Energy can be turned into matter.
C) Efficiency is the ratio of useful energy to wasted energy.
D) Energy can be dispersed through a vacuum.
E) There are always losses when energy is transformed from one type to another.

Question 27

Which of the following statements is **FALSE**?

A) A beam of light exits a pane of glass at a different angle than it entered.
B) A beam of light reflects at an angle dependent on the angle of incidence.
C) Light travels a shorter distance to reach the bottom of a pool filled with water than a pool without water.
D) Any neutrally charged atom has the potential to emit light.
E) Photons are particles without a mass.

END OF SECTION

Section 3

1) *'Doctors will eventually become obsolete as a result of advancing medical technologies.'*

Explain what this statement means. Argue to the contrary. To what extent do you agree with the statement?

2) *"Science is a procedure for testing and rejecting hypotheses, not a compendium of certain knowledge."*

Stephen Jay Gould

What do you understand from the statement above? Explain why it might be argued that science does rely on a compendium of certain knowledge? To what extent is science defined by the challenging of preconceived hypotheses?

3) *'Animal euthanasia should be made illegal'*

Explain what this statement means. Argue to the contrary that animal euthanasia should remain legal. To what extent do you agree with the statement?

4) *'The primary duty of a doctor is to prolong life as much as possible'*

What does this statement mean? Argue to the contrary, that the primary duty of a doctor is not to prolong life. To what extent do you agree with this statement?

END OF PAPER

MOCK PAPER H

Section 1

Question 1:
A chemical change may add something to a substance, or subtract something from it, or it may both subtract and add, making a new substance with entirely different properties. Sulphur and carbon are two stable solids. The chemical union of the two forms a volatile liquid. A substance may be at one time a solid, at another a liquid, at another a gas, and yet not undergo any chemical change, because in each case the chemical composition is identical.

Which of the following statements cannot be reliably concluded from the above passage?

A) The chemical composition of a compound may influence its physical nature.
B) Substances can exist as solid, liquid or gas, without their chemical composition changing.
C) Chemicals can be combined to create a new substance with similar or very different properties.
D) Combining two substances in one state can lead to the production of a compound in a completely different state.
E) The transition from solid to liquid is not a chemical one.

Question 2:
In the sequence B Y F U I R K P ? ? Which two letters come next?

A) U N   B) M N   C) L O   D) H O   E) N M

Question 3:
An insect differs from a horse, for example, as much as a modern printing press differs from the press Franklin used. Both machines are made of iron, steel, wood, etc., and both print; but the plan of their structure differs throughout, and some parts are wanting in the simpler press, which are present and absolutely essential in the other. So with the two sorts of animals; they are built up originally out of protoplasm, or the original jelly-like germinal matter, which fills the cells composing their tissues, and nearly the same chemical elements occur in both, but the mode in which these are combined, the arrangement of their products: the muscular, nervous and skin tissues, differ in the two animals.

Which of the following statements can be reliably concluded from the above passage?

A) The printing press has adapted from the press Franklin used, due to the designers observing differences in nature.
B) Horses and insects differ as they are made up of completely different chemical elements.
C) The muscular, nervous and skin tissues are what define an organism.
D) Chemical elements make up protoplasm, which is the building block for all major organisms.
E) It is the manner in which chemicals are arranged that determine an organism as a final product.

Question 4:
What day comes two days after the day, which comes four days after the day, which comes immediately after the day, which comes two days before Monday?

A) Monday   B) Tuesday   C) Thursday   D) Saturday   E) Sunday

Question 5:

Cellulose is distinguished by its inherent constructive functions, and these functions take effect in the plastic or colloidal condition of the substance. These properties are equally conspicuous in the synthetical derivatives of the compound.

Which of the following statements would weaken the above passage?

A) Cellulose has a constructive role in nature.
B) Synthetic cellulose is made from natural cellulose.
C) Synthetic and natural cellulose are structurally very similar.
D) Synthetic cellulose only actually shares some of its properties with natural cellulose.
E) Synthetics cellulose is more useful in industry than natural cellulose.

Question 6:

If John gives Michael £20, the ratio of their money is 2:1. If Michael gives John £5, the ratio of John's money to Michael's is 5:1. How much money do they have combined?

A) £180   B) £120   C) £90   D) £210   E) £150

Question 7:

From the primitive pine-torch to the paraffin candle, how wide an interval! Between them how vast a contrast! The means adopted by man to illuminate his home at night, stamp at once his position in the scale of civilisation. The fluid bitumen of the far East, blazing in rude vessels of baked earth; the Etruscan lamp, exquisite in form, yet ill adapted to its office; the whale, seal, or bear fat, filling the hut of the Esquimaux or Lap with odour rather than light; the huge wax candle on the glittering altar, the range of gas lamps in our streets, all have their stories to tell.

Which of the following statements best summarises the above passage?

A) Burning animal fat was the original way to produce fire.
B) The use of fire has spread to all corners of the Earth.
C) Using fire for light is what defines us as being human.
D) Each light source over the globe is able to tell its own tale.
E) The development and evolution of the use of fire helps to define mankind as a civilisation.

Question 8:

972 patients ordered food for lunch. They could choose roast chicken, mac and cheese, vegetable chilli or cottage pie. Half chose the roast chicken, 1/3 chose the mac and cheese and 1/12 chose the cottage pie.

How many opted for the vegetarian option?
A) 81   B) 92   C) 68   D) 95   E) 102

Question 9:

It was a little late to search for the philosophers' stone in 1669, yet it was in such a search that phosphorus was discovered. Wilhelm Homberg (1652-1715) described it in the following manner: "a man little known, of low birth, with a bizarre and mysterious nature in all he did, found this luminous matter while searching for something else."

What can be reliably concluded about the above passage?

A) Phosphorous was easy to identify as a result of its luminous nature.
B) Phosphorous was found as a result of this man's low social status.
C) Phosphorous was identified by accident, in the search for the philosophers' stone.
D) Wilhelm Homberg discovered phosphorous.
E) Phosphorous was discovered in the 18th century.

Question 10:

How many minutes past noon is it, if 3 times this many minutes before 3pm is 28 minutes later than this many minutes past noon?

A) 54   B) 32   C) 45   D) 38   E) 18

Question 11:

Everyone is familiar with the main facts of such a life-story as that of a moth or butterfly. The form of the adult insect is dominated by the wings—two pairs of scaly wings, carried respectively on the middle and hindmost of the three segments that make up the *thorax* or central region of the insect's body. Each of these three segments carries a pair of legs.

Which of the following statements can be concluded from the above statement?

A) The wings of the insects alternate patterns when the insect flies.
B) The wings that attach to the segments of the insect's body are the most prominent feature of the butterfly or moth.
C) Wings attach to each of the three segments of the thorax.
D) Moths and butterflies are very similar in that each segment of their thorax carries a pair of legs.
E) Scaly wings protect these creatures from predators.

Question 12:

John and Mary are selling cakes at a cake sale. John has 8 cupcakes and 56 brownies, where as Mary has 12 cupcakes and 24 brownies. What is the difference between the percentages of brownies in the two stalls?

A) 6%   B) 115/3%   C) 19.25%   D) 125/6%   E) 22.2%

Question 13:

In 2007 AD, Halley's Comet and Comet Encke were observed in the same calendar year. Halley's Comet is observed on average once every 73 years; Comet Encke is observed on average once every 104 years. Based on this, estimate the calendar year in which both Halley's Comet and Comet Encke are next observed in the same year.

A) 9559 AD   B) 2114 AD   C) 5643 AD   D) 3562 AD   E) 1757 AD

Question 14:

The supreme court of Judicature at Athens punished a boy for putting out the eyes of a poor bird; and parents and masters should never overlook an instance of cruelty to anything that has life, however minute, and seemingly contemptible the object may be.

Which of the following statements best summarises the above passage?
A) The boy was prosecuted because the bird is a large enough organism.
B) Putting out the eyes of an organism is the most unacceptable form of animal cruelty.
C) The more important to mankind the animal, the worse the animal cruelty crime is.
D) Any cruelty to any creature is an action that should not be tolerated.
E) It is only acceptable to harm an animal so long as it benefits a human.

Question 15:

In a school there are 40 more girls than there are boys. The boys make up a percentage of 40% of the school. What is the number of students in the school?

A) 150   B) 200   C) 300   D) 500   E) 720

Question 16:

5 cars are travelling down a road in a line. The red car is following the blue car; the yellow car is in front of the green car. The purple car is between the green car and the blue car. What colour is the car second in line?

A) Red   B) Blue   C) Yellow   D) Green   E) Purple

Question 17:

To get to school, Joanne takes the school bus every morning. If she misses this, then she can take the public bus to school. The school bus arrives at 08:15, which if she misses will come again at 08:37. The public bus comes every 17 minutes, starting at 06:56. The school bus takes 24 minutes to get to her school; the public bus takes 18 minutes. If she arrives at the bus stop at 08:25, which bus must she catch to get to school first?

A) The 08:37   B) The 08:26 public   C) The 08: 38   D) The 08: 31
    school bus   bus   public bus   public bus

Question 18:

Puddle ducks are typically birds of fresh, shallow marshes and rivers rather than of large lakes and bays. They are good divers, but usually feed by dabbling or tipping rather than submerging. The speculum, or coloured wing patch, is generally iridescent and bright, and often a tell-tale field mark. Any duck feeding in croplands will likely be a puddle duck, for most of this group are sure-footed and can walk and run well on land. Their diet is mostly vegetable, and grain-fed mallards or pintails or acorn-fattened wood ducks are highly regarded as food.

Which of the following statements summarises the above passage best?

A) Other ducks are often eaten by puddle ducks in both large lakes and shallower waters.
B) Puddle ducks feed mainly without diving to gain vegetarian food sources.
C) Puddle ducks are the most common duck seen in croplands because they are vegetarian.
D) Other ducks are prone to predate on puddle ducks.
E) Puddle ducks live in large lakes as they can access vegetable food sources easily.

Question 19:

When the earth had to be prepared for the habitation of man, a veil, as it were, of intermediate being was spread between him and its darkness, in which were joined, in a subdued measure, the stability and the insensibility of the Earth, and the passion and perishing of mankind.

Which of the following statements best summarises the above statement?

A) The veil discussed is what links the good and evil of the human race.
B) Without this veil, mankind would not exist.
C) The Earth has more good than evil.
D) The veil keeps the human race alive.
E) Mankind would be better off without such a veil.

Question 20:

What is the value of ? in the following sequence:

3 1 6 8
8 4 5 0
4 2 7 8
9 2 3 ?

A) 5   B) 4   C) 8   D) 2   E) 7

Question 21:

Metformin has been thought to inhibit the process of fat cell growth. This is because *in vitro* metformin causes fat cells to stop growing. However, when a metformin inhibitor is used alongside metformin, the fat cells still don't grow. Thus we can conclude that metformin does not inhibit fat cell growth.

Which of the following statements highlights the flaw in the argument?

A) Metformin doesn't inhibit fat cell growth.
B) The mechanism by which metformin inhibits fat cell growth is poorly understood.
C) We are not aware of how this inhibitor acts to inhibit the actions of metformin.
D) Fat cell growth has not been quantified here.
E) Metformin does not inhibit fat cell growth *in vivo*.

Question 22:

All dancers are strong. Some dancers are pretty. Alexandra is strong, and Katie is pretty.

Choose a correct statement.

A) Alexandra is a dancer
B) Katie is not a dancer
C) A dancer can be strong and pretty
D) A dancer can be strong and ugly

Question 23:

During the last fifteen years the subject of bacteriology has developed with a marvellous rapidity. At the beginning of the ninth decade of the century bacteria were scarcely heard of outside of scientific circles, and very little was known about them even among scientists. Today they are almost household words, and everyone who reads is beginning to recognise that they have important relations to everyday life.

Which of the following statements would best support the above passage?
A) Bacteriology has improved due to the advancements in our ability to see and study such organisms.
B) Bacteria are too small to see in everyday life.
C) The development of antibiotics has helped us to understand bacteria better.
D) Every household understands the problems with bacterial infections.
E) Bacteria were much scarcer in the ninth decade than they are today.

Question 24:

Read the following statements. Which of the options is correct regarding whether the conclusions drawn from the statements are true or not?

Statements:
➢ No man is a lion.
➢ Joseph is a man.

Conclusions:
➢ **I:** Joseph is not a lion.
➢ **II:** All men are not Joseph.

A) Conclusion I is TRUE and Conclusion II is TRUE
B) Conclusion I is TRUE and FALSE
C) Conclusion I is TRUE and Conclusion II is CAN'T TELL
D) Conclusion I is FALSE and Conclusion II is CAN'T TELL
E) Conclusion I is FALSE and Conclusion II is TRUE

Question 25:

We may define a food as any substance, which will repair the functional waste of the body, increase its growth, or maintain the heat, muscular, and nervous energy. In its most comprehensive sense, the oxygen of the air is a food; as although it is admitted by the lungs, it passes into the blood, and there re-acts upon the other food, which has passed through the stomach. It is usual, however, to restrict the term food to such nutriment as enters the body by the intestinal canal. Water is often spoken of as being distinct from food, but for this there is no sufficient reason.

Which of the following statements highlights the weakness in the passage?
A) Oxygen also is absorbed in the digestive tract.
B) Water is only made up of two elements, which is why it is not classified as food.
C) Water is needed for bodily functions and therefore must be food.
D) It is not explained why water is not classified as a food.
E) Any substance that is involved in a physiological process must have originated from food.

Question 26:

Billy is James's father. 4 years ago, Billy's age was 4 times that of James. After 6 years, the ages of the Billy and James are in the ratio of 5:2. How old is Billy?

A) 12   B) 13   C) 14   D) 15   E) 16

Question 27:
The word soap appears to have been originally applied to the product obtained by treating tallow with ashes. In its strictly chemical sense it refers to combinations of fatty acids with metallic bases, a definition which includes not only sodium stearate, oleate and palmitate, which form the bulk of the soaps of commerce, but also the linoleates of lead, manganese, etc., used as driers, and various pharmaceutical preparations, *e.g.*, mercury oleate, zinc oleate and lead plaster, together with a number of other metallic salts of fatty acids.

What can be reliably concluded about the above passage?

A) All metallic salts of fatty acids are classified as soaps.
B) Soaps are only used in industry for commercial use, driers and as pharmaceutical preparations.
C) Treating tallow with acids forms a soap as it results in fatty acids combining with a metallic acid.
D) All soaps are fatty acids combined with metallic bases.
E) All metals form soaps used in industry.

Question 28:
The average marks scored by 12 students is 73. If the scores of Bea, Bay and Boe are included, the average becomes 73.6. If Bea scored 68 marks and Boe scored 6 more than Bay, what was Bay's score?

A) 75   B) 76   C) 77   D) 78   E) 79

Question 29:
A building company employs 90 men to work for 8 hours per day to complete some building work. The company wants to finish work in 200 days but after 120 days, the work is only a third complete. If the men start working 12-hour days, how many more men are required to complete the work on time?

A) 170   B) 180   C) 190   D) 200   E) 210

Question 30:
The organs that form the digestive tract are the mouth, pharynx, oesophagus, stomach, intestines and the annexed glands, viz.: the salivary, liver, and pancreas. The development of these organs differs in the different species of animals. For example, solipeds possess a small, simple stomach and capacious, complicated intestines. Just the opposite is true of ruminants. The different species of ruminants possess a large, complicated stomach, and comparatively simple intestines. In swine we meet with a more highly developed stomach than that of solipeds and a more simple intestinal tract. Of all domestic animals the most simple digestive tract occurs in the dog.

What can be reliably concluded from the above passage?

A) Dogs have the simplest digestive tracts of domesticated animals due to their size.
B) Solipeds and ruminants differ only in their digestive tracts.
C) The more complex the digestive tract, the more complex the organism.
D) Mammals have varying digestive tracts that are adapted for their environments.
E) The mammalian digestive tract is vital for the survival of the animal.

Question 31:
If every alternative letter starting from A of the English alphabet is written in lower case, and the rest are all written in upper case, how would the day "Wednesday" be written?

A) wEdNEsdAy   C) WEdnESdAY   E) WedNesdAY
B) weDNesDay   D) weDneSDaY

Question 32:
A man covers a distance in 1hr 24min by covering 2/3 of the distance at 4 km/h and the rest at 5km/h. What distance does he cover?

A) 5km   B) 6km   C) 7km   D) 8km

END OF SECTION

Section 2

Question 1:

Hydrogen Bicarbonate (HCO_3^-) acts as a buffer in the blood i.e. to keep the PH close to 7.

Which statement is true regarding bicarbonate?

A) It is alkaline.
B) It is an acidic molecule.
C) If the pH of the blood drops below 7, bicarbonate will release the H^+ ion to stabilise the pH.
D) It is only released when the pH drops below 7.
E) It is bound to protein in the blood.

Question 2:

Which of the statements regarding this series circuit is true?

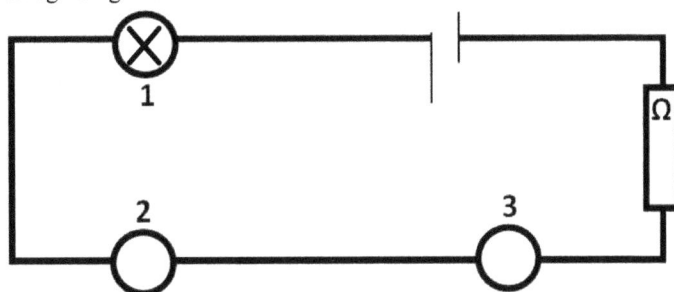

A) Current is different at different points in the circuit.
B) Potential difference is shared between the three lightbulbs.
C) Resistance is constant throughout the circuit.
D) The current is higher in bulb 1 than in bulbs 2 and 3.

Question 3:

Consider the equations: A: $y = 3x$ and B: $y = 6/x - 7$. At what values of x do the two equations intersect?

A) x=2 and x=9   C) x=6 and x=27   E) x=18
B) x=3 and x=6   D) x=6

Question 4:

Bill wants to lay down laminate flooring in his living room, which has an in-built circular fish tank that he will have to lay the flooring around. He has decided to buy planks that he can cut to fit the dimensions of his room. He must, however, buy whole planks and cut them down himself. The room's dimensions are given below, as are those of one plank.

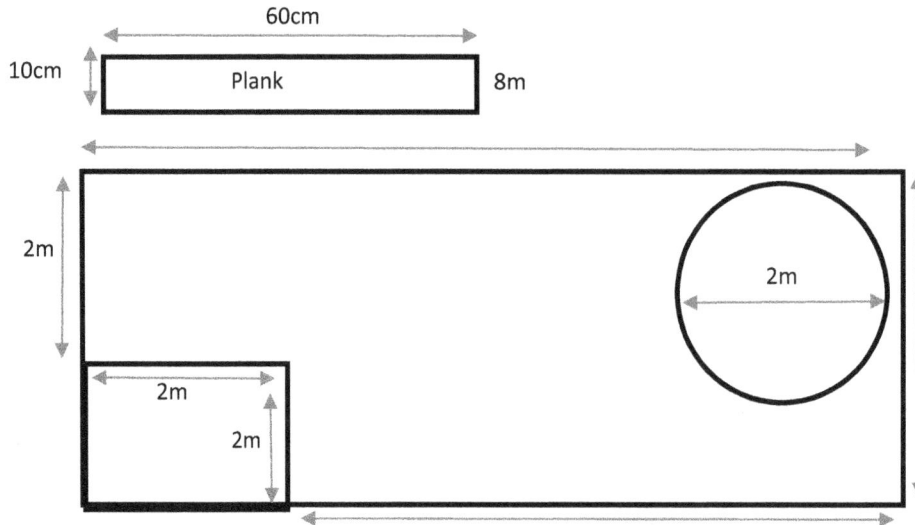

Calculate the number of planks needed to cover the whole floor. Take $\pi = 3$.

A) 30   B) 417   C) 600   D) 589   E) 43

Question 5:

In pregnancy the foetus is supplied with blood from the mother via the umbilical cord. This cord is comprised of one vein and two arteries. The table below shows which vessel carries which type of blood in which direction.

	Vessel	Direction	Blood
1.	Vein	Mother to foetus	Oxygenated
2.	Artery	Foetus to Mother	Deoxygenated
3.	Artery	Foetus to Mother	Oxygenated
4.	Vein	Mother to Foetus	Deoxygenated

Which options are correct?

A) 1 only   C) 3 only   E) 1 and 2   G) 4 and 1
B) 2 only   D) 4 only   F) 2 and 3   H) 3 and 1

Question 6:

Solve $y = x^2 - 3x + 4$ and $y - x = 1$ as (x,y).

A) (-1, 2) and (3,4)   C) (7,-2) and (6,5)   E) (1,-1) and (-7,-1)
B) (1,2) and (3,4)   D) (2,-3) and (4,-1)

Question 7:

Calculate the radius of a sphere which has a surface area three times as great as its volume.

A) 0.5   D) 2
B) 1   E) 2.5
C) 1.5   F) More information is needed

Question 8:

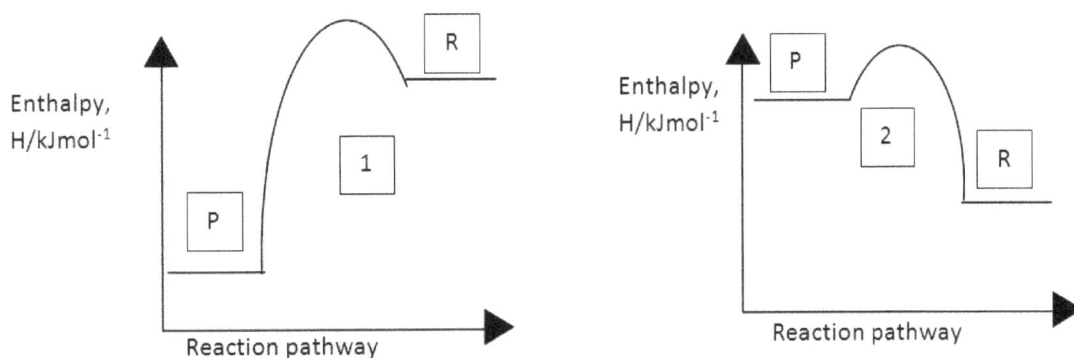

The two graphs shown above are Enthalpy profile diagrams. Which best describes an endothermic reaction?

	Graph	ΔH	Heat energy	Stability of reactants
A)	1	Negative	Absorbed from surroundings	P is more stable than R
B)	2	Negative	Released to surroundings	R is more stable than P
C)	1	Positive	Absorbed from surroundings	P is more stable than R
D)	2	Positive	Absorbed from surroundings	R is more stable than P

Question 9:

What is the function of the kidneys?

1. Ultrafiltration
2. Kill bacteria in the blood
3. Reabsorption
4. Release of waste
5. Store water
6. Produce hormones
7. Blood glucose regulation

A) 1 only   C) 3 only   E) 5 only   G) 3 and 5   I) 4, 5 and 6

B) 2 only   D) 4 only   F) 6 and 7   H) 1, 3 and 4

Question 10:

Mike and Vanessa are two healthy adults. They have two children. Their first child, Rory, was born with Haemophilia B, an X linked recessive disorder that causes problems with blood clotting. They have just had another baby, a girl and want to get her tested for the condition. What is the likelihood of the baby girl having the condition?

A) 0%   B) 25%   C) 50%   D) 75%   E) 34%

Question 11:

Pyrite, also known as Fool's Gold, is an ore of Iron containing sulphur in the form of iron (II) disulphide, FeS_2. By mass 75% of this ore is FeS_2.

Calculate the maximum mass of iron that can be extracted from 480kg of ore.
[A_r: Fe = 55; S = 32]

A) 167.7kg   B) 200kg   C) 360.5kg   D) 118kg   E) 120.2kg

Question 12:

$X_{(s)} + FeSO_{4(aq)} \rightarrow XSO_{4(aq)} + Fe_{(S)}$

Which metal can be correctly be substituted in X's place?

A) Tin (Sn)   C) Lead (Pb)   E) Copper (Cu)
B) Zinc (Zn)   D) Silver (Ag)

Question 13:

Which of the following statements is true regarding Red Shift?

A) The further a distant galaxy or celestial object is, the further down the red end of the light spectrum it's light will be.
B) The closer a galaxy gets, the longer it's wavelengths get, thus moving down the red end of the spectrum.
C) Red shift means that we never see the real light from distant galaxies.
D) We can never tell how far away galaxies are using red shift.

Question 14:

Which is true regarding X-rays?

A) X-rays do not pass through denser materials like bone and that's why they show up as white on the X-ray film.
B) X-rays pass through bone but not skin and soft tissue, and that's why bones show up white on the X-ray film.
C) X-rays don't ionise cells and thus are safe.
D) Gamma rays are safer than X-rays.

Question 15:

Rearrange $\frac{(16x+11)}{(4x+5)} = 4y^2 + 2$ to make x the subject

A) $x = \frac{20y^2-1}{[16-4\,(4y^2+2)]}$ C) $= \frac{6y^2-1}{[16-4\,(4y^2+2)]}$ E) $= \frac{7y^2-1}{[6-14\,(6+7)]}$

B) $= \frac{20y^2-8}{[16-6\,(4y^2+2)]}$ D) $= \frac{21y^2-1}{[16-4\,(2y^2+2)]}$

Question 16:

The element shown below is Germanium. It has an ionic charge of 4+. How many electrons does one atom of Germanium have?

73
Ge
32

A) 32   B) 73   C) 36   D) 41   E) 4

Question 17:

Bacteria invade the body and produce toxins that kill cells.

What are some of the first line defences the body has to prevent bacteria entering?
1. Mucus lining the airways
2. Heat produced by the body
3. Skin
4. Antibodies produced by the immune system
5. Toxins produced by the body
6. Hydrochloric acid in the stomach

A) 1 only
B) 2 only
C) 3 only

D) 1, 3, 4 and 6
E) 4, 5 and 6
F) 1, 3 and 6

G) 2 and 4

Question 18:

If $(3p + 5)^2 = 24p + 49$, calculate p.

A) -5 or -9   B) -3 or -6   C) -4 or 6   D) -6 or 4   E) 4 or -2

Question 19:

Reaction rates are explained by the Collision Theory. This theory states that particles have to collide (hard enough) in order to react.

Which of the statements below are true?
1. An increase in the temperature of the system can cause more collisions with greater force, therefore causing more reactions.
2. Smaller particles are don't collide or react as well.
3. Increasing the pressure of the system does not cause more collisions.
4. The collision theory only applies to gasses.
5. Increasing the surface area of the reactant increases the chances of collision.

A) 1 only
B) 2 only

C) 3 only
D) 4 only

E) 2 and 3
F) 3, 4 and 5

G) 1 and 5

Question 20:

When someone is lost in the mountains, the rescue team often wraps an aluminium covered plastic sheet around them in order to keep them warm.

Which of the statements are true regarding the effects on heat loss may have on their body?
1. There is less heat loss through conduction.
2. Air is trapped closer to the body and this means that there is less heat loss due to convection.
3. Aluminium absorbs more sunlight and thus this keeps the person warm as more heat is absorbed.

A) 1 only
B) 2 only

C) 3 only
D) 1 and 2

E) 1, 2, 3
F) 2 and 3

G) None

Question 21:

Which of the following is true with regards to osmosis?

A) It does not require a concentration gradient
B) It can apply to any substance, not just water
C) It is the movement of water across a partially permeable membrane
D) It is an active process
E) Transporters move water molecules across the membrane of cells

Question 22

For the following reaction, which of the statements is true?

$$CH_{4(g)} + 2O_{2(g)} \rightarrow 2H_2O_{(aq)} + CO_{2(g)}$$

A) This is an example of complete combustion.
B) By increasing the concentration of CO_2 you can increase the rate of combustion
C) The reaction is anaerobic
D) Combustion of a gas always produces a liquid like water
E) If you remove some of the oxygen you get more product.

Question 23:

Which of the following is a unit of resistance?

A) $V.A^{-1}$ B) $C.A$ C) $C.\Omega$ D) $V.\Omega^{-1}$ E) $W.V^{-1}$ F) J

Question 24:

To screw a piece of wood into a plank of wood, Bob uses a 20cm spanner. The moment of the force used to twist the screw into the plank is 40Nm. How much force does Bob need to exert on the screw?

A) 2   B) 0.2   C) 80   D) 200   E) 0.5   F) 820

Question 25:

The carbon cycle is the cycle regarding the intake and release of carbon by organisms. Which of these statements are true?

A) Plants take carbon via photosynthesis and taking nutrients from the soil, which have come from decayed organisms.
B) Animals give off carbon via respiration, waste, eating and death.
C) The CO_2 in the air comes from burning of plant/animal products and respiration from living organisms only.
D) Trees do not store any carbon as they give it all off as carbon dioxide.

Question 26:

Refraction occurs when a wave passes from a material of low density to a material of high density or vice versa.

Which of these statements regarding refraction is true?
A) If a wave hits a different medium at an angle, the wave does not change direction.
B) If a wave hits a boundary face on, it slows down but carries on in the same direction. Thus it has a shorter wavelength but the same frequency.
C) Waves can be refracted even if they hit the boundary head on.
D) Light is the only type of wave that can be refracted.
E) Glass to air slows down the wave.

Question 27:

Enzymes are thought to work by two mechanisms – lock and key or the induced fit theory. The Lock and Key theory states that the active site of an enzyme is already perfectly shaped for the substrate, whereas the induced fit theory states that the enzyme's active site moulds itself around the substrate's shape. Which of these statements is true?

A) Enzymes are substrate specific.
B) The induced fit theory allows multiple, different types of substrates to be acted on by one enzyme.
C) The induced fit theory allows multiple, different types of enzymes to work on the same substrate.
D) The lock and key theory does not allow space for catatonic reactions (breaking the substrate up.

END OF SECTION

Section 3

1) *"Time and time again, throughout the history of medical practice, what was once considered as "scientific" eventually becomes regarded as "bad practice"."* - **David Stewart**

What does this statement mean? Give some examples of times when scientific practice has become bad practice and describe how this has had an impact on medicine.

2) *"Formerly, when religion was strong and science was weak, men mistook magic for medicine; now, when science is strong and religion is weak, men mistake medicine for magic."* – **Thomas Szasz**

What does this statement mean? Do you think it is correct in assuming all men mistake medicine for magic?

3) *'Approximately 26.9% of the adult population in the UK is obese. We should be offering bariatric surgery to every obese person that walks through the doors.'*

Explain what this statement means. Argue to the contrary. To what extent do you agree with the statement?

4) *'Placebos may solve the problem of patients demanding medication they do not need.'*

Explain what this statement means. Argue the contrary. To what extent do you agree with the statement?

END OF PAPER

ANSWERS

ANSWER KEY

	Paper E		Paper F		Paper G		Paper H	
	Section 1	Section 2	Section 1	Section 2	Section 1	Section 2	Section 1	Section 2
1	C	1 D	1 D	1 G	1 C	1 B	1 A	1 A
2	D	2 E	2 A	2 D	2 D	2 H	2 C	2 B
3	C	3 C	3 C	3 C	3 B	3 D	3 E	3 C
4	A	4 A	4 D	4 D	4 E	4 E	4 D	4 B
5	B	5 B	5 A	5 C	5 C	5 B	5 D	5 E
6	D	6 D	6 B	6 C	6 C	6 D	6 E	6 B
7	C	7 F	7 E	7 A	7 B	7 A	7 E	7 B
8	B	8 A	8 E	8 A	8 B	8 B	8 A	8 C
9	E	9 F	9 D	9 C	9 B	9 A	9 C	9 H
10	A	10 C	10 B	10 B	10 A	10 A	10 D	10 A
11	C	11 D	11 A	11 A	11 B	11 D	11 B	11 A
12	B	12 B	12 D	12 C	12 E	12 B	12 D	12 B
13	C	13 C	13 C	13 H	13 D	13 F	13 A	13 A
14	E	14 E	14 A	14 B	14 C	14 E	14 D	14 A
15	D	15 B	15 E	15 C	15 E	15 E	15 B	15 A
16	E	16 C	16 D	16 D	16 A	16 B	16 D	16 A
17	A	17 E	17 B	17 E	17 B	17 B	17 C	17 F
18	D	18 F	18 B	18 C	18 E	18 D	18 B	18 D
19	E	19 A	19 A	19 A	19 C	19 B	19 A	19 G
20	E	20 B	20 B	20 B	20 E	20 C	20 E	20 E
21	D	21 F	21 B	21 A	21 B	21 B	21 C	21 C
22	B&E	22 B	22 E	22 D	22 C	22 D	22 C	22 A
23	D	23 D	23 D	23 B	23 D	23 D	23 A	23 A
24	C	24 E	24 D	24 C	24 A	24 C	24 C	24 D
25	B	25 E	25 B	25 C	25 E	25 C	25 D	25 B
26	C	26 D	26 A	26 D	26 C	26 E	26 C	26 B
27	C	27 B	27 D	27 C	27 D	27 A	27 D	27 A
28	A		28 B		28 B		28 C	
29	A		29 A		29 D		29 B	
30	D		30 E		30 D		30 D	
31	A		31 C		31 C		31 B	
32	A		32 B		32 D		32 B	

Raw to Scaled Scores

Section 1							Section 2					
1	1	11	2.8	21	5.4	31	8.3	1	1	11	3.5	21	6.6
2	1	12	3.0	22	5.7	32	9	2	1	12	3.7	22	6.9
3	1	13	3.2	23	6.0			3	1.3	13	4	23	7.3
4	1	14	3.5	24	6.3			4	1.6	14	4.3	24	7.6
5	1.2	15	3.7	25	6.6			5	1.9	15	4.6	25	8
6	1.5	16	4.0	26	6.9			6	2.2	16	5	26	8.5
7	1.8	17	4.2	27	7.1			7	2.5	17	5.3	27	9
8	2.0	18	4.5	28	7.4			8	2.8	18	5.6		
9	2.3	19	4.8	29	7.7			9	3.0	19	5.9		
10	2.5	20	5.1	30	8.0			10	3.2	20	6.2		

MOCK PAPER E ANSWERS

Section 1

Question 1: C

In this question we are asked to find a conclusion for the passage. The passage discusses how some birds fly north to breed as there is the conditions are better suited to them and they only have to travel a few miles to gather food. Thus it is fair to conclude that the reason for these birds migration is because the food and conditions are more suited to them, therefore the answer is C.

Question 2: D

X is married to A who is a lawyer, so B and C are either a doctor or a lawyer respectively. Y is not married to an engineer, and C is not a doctor so Y must be married to B who is a doctor, and Z must be married to C who is an engineer, so the correct answer is D, as none of these options are available.

Question 3: C

The passage says nothing about whether it is more important to have good doctor-patient relations than scientific progress, so answer E) is not a valid conclusion. Answer D) is a direct argument against the question, which claims the naming system *should* be changed, so answer D) is not a conclusion. The passage states that the confusing system causes problems in scientific literature, but this does *not* necessarily mean that changing it would allow faster progress in scientific research, so answer B) is not a valid conclusion. Answers A) and C) are both valid points from the passage, but we can see that Answer A) is a *reason* stated in the passage, which helps support the statement in C). Thus, Answer C) is the main conclusion.

Question 4: A

Answers B) and E) are both in contradiction with stated points in the question, which states that there is now powerful evidence human bodies *are* set up for long-distance running, and that it is well established that humans evolved in Africa. Answer C) is irrelevant, because the presence of other theories does *not* necessarily affect whether we should believe this theory based on the new evidence. Answer D) actually strengthens the argument, suggesting that the new evidence does provide powerful reasons to believe this theory. Answer A) however is a valid flaw, that evidence supporting a theory does not necessarily *prove* that it is true. Thus, the answer is A).

Question 5: B

There is a 3l and 5l bucket – therefore 4 litres can be measured from the difference between the buckets as follows. Fill the 5l bucket, decant 3l into the smaller bucket and then you are left with 2l in the large bucket. Pour this into the tank. Repeat the process again, decanting the remaining 2l into the tank once again to make 4l in total. The first time, 5 litres was required. The second time, the 3 litres from the second bucket could be tipped back into the 5l bucket, and then filled up with fresh water to measure the final 2 litres in. Therefore 4 + 3 = 7 litres of water is sufficient to fill the tank with 4l.

Question 6: D

To answer this question, make a timeline showing the locations of the different genres of books. Place each book on the timeline as appropriate, making sure to indicate where more than one location is a possibility. From that, you will see that literature books are located to the right of engineering. This is true since they are to the right of art (which we know is right of mathematics (and therefore engineering, since the run between the sciences is uninterrupted)). The other statements, whilst potentially true, cannot be deduced for certain.

Question 7: C

The passage tells us that brand new cars lose value quickly, despite the car being virtually unchanged. Therefore in the absence of any contradictory information, it is reasonable to conclude that buying second hand cars is a wise choice.

Question 8: B

First, calculate how many bottles are sold. 2000 – (2000x0.9x0.8) = 560 bottles. Then divide the total profit by the number of units to give the profit per unit, which comes to 11200/560 = £20 per bottle.

Question 9: E

The definition of timelessness requires something to be tested by time. Something that modern furniture cannot fulfil. Therefore statement E expresses a significant flaw in the reasoning. The other statements do not refer to the 'timelessness' aspect of furniture, therefore they are not directly relevant to the argument.

Question 10: A

The passage talks about the benefits of drinking red wine, not about living near to vineyards. The passage does not state that Italians drink more wine than Germans, therefore the assumption that they do is central to the argument.

Question 11: C

Tom arrives at 1620, and leaves 45 mins after Jane leaves. Therefore he also leaves 45 mins after Hannah leaves, since Jane and Hannah leave together. Since his journey is 10 mins faster than Hannah's, he arrives only 35 minutes after Hannah arrives (which happens to be 1620). Therefore Hannah arrives 35 minutes earlier than this, at 1545. Since she left at 1430, her journey took 75 minutes. Jane's journey took 40% longer (1.4 x 75 = 105 minutes). Therefore leaving at the same time as Hannah, 1430, Jane arrived 105 minutes later at 1615.

Question 12: B

This is a simultaneous equations question. Let x be the number of standard tickets sold, and y be the number of premium tickets sold.

Therefore: $x + y = 600$; $10x + 16y = 6,600$

$x = 600 - y$ » substitute: $10(600 - y) + 16y = 6600$

$6y = 600$

$y = 100$, therefore 100 premium tickets were sold.

Question 13: C

Between 20th January and 23rd May, there are 123 days. In 123 days, the moon makes 123/28 = 4.39 orbits. This is equal to 4.39 x 360° = 1580°

Question 14: E

You are looking for a strong opposition to the proposition that students at drama academies are not taught well academically. The strongest opposition would be evidence that such students perform academically well in some objective measure. Evidence of significantly above average GCSE results provides this.

Question 15: D

You should definitely draw this one out on paper. Trace out the paths and you find that both people have a net displacement of 11km to the North. Therefore since Anil is only net 2km East, and Suresh is 17km East of the starting point, there is a 15km separation between them

Question 16: E

If three times the final amount of concrete is ground off by the builder, three quarters of the original thickness is removed, hence one quarter remains. 14/4 = 3.5cm

Question 17: A

Walking at 4mph, 3 miles takes ¾ hour = 45 mins. Adding the 5 minute stop, Chris will arrive at 1820, since he set off at 1730. At 24mph, 6 miles takes ¼ hour, 15 mins. Therefore setting off at 1810, Sarah will arrive at Laura's at 1825. Therefore Chris arrives 5 minutes earlier than Sarah.

Question 18: D

The passage tells us that illegal downloads are causing harm to the music industry. Whilst it gives an example, this does not mean the stated example is the principal issue. The conclusion that best fits the passage as a whole is to say illegal downloading is more harmful than many people think, given their willingness to undertake it.

Question 19: E

First, calculate the amount of water needed for each type of fire. Use algebra:

Use x as the amount of water used to extinguish a house fire. 40,000L = 2x , so x = 20,000L. Then, take y as the amount of water needed to extinguish a garden fire, so 70,000L = 2x + 3y. 30,000L = 3y, y= 10,000L.

Knowing this, A is correct, B is correct, C is correct and D is correct. Only E is false.

Three house and ten garden fires require 160,000 litres to extinguish, not 140,000.

Question 20: E

To answer this question, we need to use SUVAT equations, specifically:

$s = \frac{1}{2} (u + v) t$ and $s = vt + (1/2a \times t^2)$

We can calculate the distance the car initially moves before accelerating by $20ms^{-1} \times 30s = 600m$. Using the $s = vt + (1/2 a \times t^2)$, substitute in the values we know to find the distance travelled during the acceleration.

$s = 20 \times 5 + (1/2 \times 2 \times 25) = 125m$

We can calculate our new speed after the moment of acceleration by:

$20 + (5 \times 2) = 30ms^{-1}$, and the distance travelled at this new velocity by $20 \times 30 = 600m$

The distance travelled during the deceleration is found by:

$s = \frac{1}{2} (30+0) t$, as the car is coming to the stop so the final velocity is 0.

We find t by doing $30ms^{-1} / 3ms^{-2} = 10s$

So, substituting this in give the distance = 150m. Add all these distances together to give the final distance covered = 1475m.

Question 21: D

The passage only talks about people's opinions on the scheme, and not about any action which could potentially be taken. Therefore the best summary is to say that more people oppose the scheme than support it.

Question 22: B + E

The question asks for two responses, therefore you must mark two and get them both correct for one mark. The suggestion is made that reducing wild fishing will improve fish populations. This assertion carries two major assumptions – that the fishing originally caused the decline, and that the decline is reversible, and can therefore recover if the threat is removed. Select these two responses for a mark.

Question 23: D

To calculate this, you need to work out how many possible combinations there are, and how many of them contain exactly two heads. Since there are 2 possibilities and 5 trials, the number of potential outcomes is $2^5 = 32$. For two heads, any combination of two coins can show heads – and since there are 5 coins tossed, there are 10 possible combinations of exactly two heads. Therefore the probability is $^{10}/_{32}$, which is equivalent to $^5/_{16}$.

Question 24: C

For a 5 litre bucket with a 2% margin for error, the maximum possible volume is 1.02 x 5 = 5.10l, and the minimum is 0.98 x 5 = 4.90l. Therefore there is a 200ml difference between the maximum and minimum volume possible. Therefore the range of cleaning powder required is 0.2 x 40 = 8g.

Question 25: B

To calculate the cost of the call, you need to first work out its duration in minutes and multiply by the off-peak rate per minute. Then you add on the connection fee of 18p. A call of 1.4 hours = 1 hour 24 minutes = 84 mins. (84 x 22 =1848 = £18.48). £18.48 + 18p = £18.66.

Question 26: C

The passage tells us about the risks of sunbathing, and that many people do not see the danger in it. The final sentence shows us that the conclusion is a wide-ranging one, not a specific observation about UV radiation. Therefore Answer C is correct, it best sums up the passage as a whole.

Question 27: C

First calculate the total pay, then divide this by the number of hours Jim works for an hourly rate. Total pay = 3 x 8 = £24 covers the total pay for the 8 houses. Total time taken to wash all the windows = (11 windows x 8 x 2mins per window) + (15mins to pack up and walk to the next house x 7) = 281 minutes = 4.68 hours. [the total time is equal to the number of windows in total multiplied by the time taken to clean each window, plus the time travelling between the houses, which is 15 multiplied by the 7 journeys required].

Once you have worked out the number of hours Jim worked, you can find the hourly rate by £24/4.68hours = £5.12per hour.

Question 28: A

The passage argues that bottled water is pointless, as is almost identical to tap water. If bottled water had an additional benefit, such as being good for health, it might be that it makes sense to drink bottled water.

Question 29: A

Be careful – this sentence contains a triple negative. If the sentence read "...nor any cyclists that are marathon runners", it would be clear that no cyclists run marathons too. Changing the sentence to "...nor NO cyclists that AREN'T marathon runners" introduces a double negative, hence the meaning is not changed. Therefore it still means no cyclists run marathons, hence **A** is true.

Question 30: D

Draw this one out on a line. You will see that whilst we know Oakton is East of Langham, we cannot conclude its whereabouts in relation to Frampton – it could be either East or West. Therefore **D** cannot be said with certainty.

Question 31: A

Firstly calculate the surface area of the dome, then divide by the surface area covered by one pot to calculate the number of pots needed. A dome is half a sphere, so the area is given by $\frac{4\pi r^2}{2} = 12 \, x \frac{49}{2} = 294$. Since one pot covers $12m^2$, 24.5 pots are required to cover the whole dome, therefore 25 must be purchased.

Question 32: A

25 Pots x 2 Litres per pot = 50 litres of paint.

This gives a solid volume of 50 x 0.4 = 20 when the paint dries = $0.02m^3$.

The volume of the hemisphere is: $\frac{\frac{4}{3}\pi r^3}{2} = \frac{4r^3}{2}$

$= 2 \, x \, 7^3 = 686$

Hence the overall percentage decrease is: $\frac{0.02}{686} x100$

$= \frac{2}{686} = \frac{1}{343}$ 0.0029%

END OF SECTION

Section 2

Question 1: D

Firstly, convert Litres → m^3: 950 Litres = 0.95 m^3

Buoyancy Force = Volume x Density x g.

= 0.95 x 1000 x 10 = 9,500 N

Weight of the boat = mg= 600 x 10 = 6,000 N

Since buoyancy force > Weight, the boat will float.

The difference between Buoyancy Force + weight = 9500 – 6000 = 3,500N

Hence adding mass of 350kg (=3,500N as *g* is 10) will balance both forces.

Adding further mass will cause the boat to sink. Hence, the answer is 355kg (350kg won't cause sinking – merely balance the force).

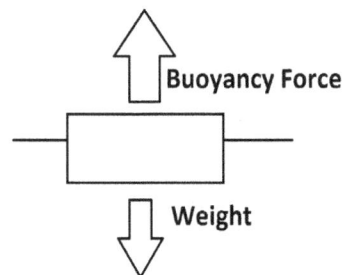

Question 2: E

Recall that reduction is the gain of electrons whilst oxidation is a loss. Also remember that oxidation the gain of oxygen, while reduction is loss. Only Iodine is gaining electrons and so shows reduction.

Question 3: C

The formula for calculating compound interest can be given as investment x (interest rate^{years}) or in short hand for this situation: $1687.5 = 500x^3$. Therefore, in order to calculate the interest rate the above formula must be rearranged to $\sqrt[3]{1687.5/500} = 1.5$ revealing an interest rate of 50%.

Question 4: A

Remember that you can separate the vertical and horizontal components of both bullets. Both bullets actually have zero vertical velocity at t=0. Thus, only gravity affects them- and it does so equally. Therefore, rather counter-intuitively, they hit the floor at the same time.

Question 5: B

To win one game, Rupert must win one squash game and one tennis game. In order to calculate the probability one winning one game, it is necessary to add the probability of winning one tennis game and losing one squash game to the probability of losing one tennis game and winning one squash game. The following calculation must be performed: $(\frac{3}{4} \times \frac{2}{3}) + (\frac{1}{4} \times \frac{1}{3}) = \frac{7}{12}$

Question 6: D

Blood flow to the kidneys is constant - not exercise dependent. Overall cardiac output increases since heart rate and stroke volume increase (because there is greater oxygen demand from exercising muscle). There is more blood flow to the muscles to fuel them and to the skin to help lose excess heat. Blood flow to the gut decreases to increase availability to muscles. Blood flow to vital organs such as the kidney and brain remains constant.

Question 7: F

To balance the equation, start working from what you're given – the oxygen. Since you know there are 15 oxygen atoms on the right, there must be the same on the left. Therefore **w** = 5. You also know that there are 30 Hydrogen atoms on the right hand side, and so you can work out x. 30-5 leaves 25 atoms unaccounted for, so x=25.

Question 8: A

Since A-T and C-G are the DNA base pairings, 29.6% Adenine implies 29.6% Thymine as well. Therefore the remaining 100 – 59.2 = 40.8% is shared between Guanine and Cytosine equally, so there is 20.4% cytosine.

Question 9: F

Structure A is the right semi-lunar valve, the pulmonary valve. It opens in systole to allow flow of blood from the right ventricle into the pulmonary artery and to the lungs. It closes in diastole to ensure the right ventricle fills only from the right atrium, maintaining a one-way flow of blood. Therefore F is true, it opens when the right atrium is emptying. None of the other statements are true.

Question 10: C

Since CO binds to the oxygen binding site of haemoglobin, it reduces oxygen binding and therefore oxygen carrying capacity of blood. Hence, the blood becomes less oxygenated. Since more blood needs to flow to deliver the same amount of oxygen, this must be accomplished by an increased in heart rate. Haemoglobin does not become heavier as the CO binds **instead** of oxygen rather than in **addition** to. Carbon Dioxide is carried in plasma so is unaffected by carbon monoxide poisoning which affects haemoglobin.

Question 11: D

A Moment of force = Force x Perpendicular distance to pivot

If the lifting arm is a uniform 5m long, the weight exerts $2000 \, x \, 10 \, x \, 5 \; = \; 100,000 \, Nm$ of torque. In addition, there is a $250 \, x \, 10 \, x \, 2.5 \; = \; 6,250 \, Nm$ contribution from the weight of the beam ($\frac{5}{7}$ the mass, acting through the centre of mass of the beam).

On the other side, the remaining $\frac{2}{7}$ of the beam makes a $100 \, x \, 10 \, x \, 1 \; = \; 1,000 \, Nm$ contribution.

Therefore, the counterbalance must make a $(100,000 \; + \; 6,250) - 1,000 \; = \; 105,250 \, Nm$ contribution. As the counterbalance arm is 2 m long, this requires a weight of $\frac{105,250}{2} \; = \; 52,625 \, N$ weight, or a mass of 5,263 kg.

The crane's height is a distracter and not needed for this question

Question 12: B

Work out the total energy transferred - 20 x 50W =1,000W of overall power by the 20 strings of lights when on. As W = Js⁻¹, can use the time the lights are on to find the energy used over this time period. 8pm – 6am is 10 hours, so in seconds is 10x60x60 = 36,000s. When multiplying this by the power of all sets of lights, gives the energy used as:

1000 W x 36,000 s = 36,000,000 J of energy, or 36,000kJ. Multiply this by 20 to account for the lights being on for 20 days = gives 720,000 kJ

As 100 kJ of energy costs 2p, need to do 720,000/100 = 7,200. Multiply this by 2p = 14,400p. Convert to pounds by dividing by 100 = **£144.**

Question 13: C

The formula for the sum of internal angles in a regular polygon is given by: $180(n-2)$, where n is the number of sides of the polygon.

Thus: $180(n-2) \; = \; 150 \, x \, n$

$180n - 360 \; = \; 150n$

$3n \; = \; 36$

$n \; = \; 12$

Each side is 15cm so the perimeter is 12 x 15cm = 180cm.

Question 14: E

For Resistors in parallel, $\frac{1}{R_T} = \frac{R_1 \, x \, R_2 \dots}{R_1 + R_2 \dots}$

For the first segment: $\frac{1}{R} = \frac{1}{Z} + \frac{1}{Z} = \frac{2}{Z}$

For the second segment: $\frac{1}{R} = \frac{1}{Z} + \frac{1}{Z} + \frac{1}{Z} = \frac{3}{Z}$

For the third segment: R = Z

Thus the total resistance is: $Z + \frac{Z}{2} + \frac{Z}{3} \; = \; 22.$

$\frac{6Z + 3Z + 2Z}{6} \; = \; 22$

$11Z \; = \; 22 \, x \, 6$

$Z \; = \; \frac{132}{11} \; = \; 12M\Omega$

Question 15: B

The volume of candle burned in 0.5 hour = $0.5 \ x \ (\pi \ x \ 2^2) \ = \ 6cm^{-3}$

$6cm^{-3} = 6 \ x \ 10^{-3} \ m^3$

Since $Density = \frac{mass}{volume}$, in this case $900 \ kgm^{-3} = \frac{mass}{6 \ x \ 10^{-3} \ m^3}$

Thus, Mass burned = $900 \ x \ 6 \ x \ 10^{-3} \ = \ 5400 \ x \ 10^{-3} kg = 5.4 \ g$

The Mr of $C_{24}H_{52}$ = $12 \ x \ 24 \ + \ 52 \ x \ 1 \ = \ 340.$

Thus the number of moles burned = $\frac{5.4}{340} \ = \ 0.016 \ moles.$

Total Energy transferred = $0.016 \ x \ 11,000$

$= \ 16 \ x \ 10^{-3} \ x \ 11 \ x \ 10^3 = 11 \ x \ 16$

$= \ 176 \ kJ \ = \ 175,000 \ J$

Question 16: C

$250 \ kJ \ = \ 25 \ x \ 10^4 \ J$

$25 \ x \ 10^4 \ J \ = \ \frac{25 \ x 10^4}{4.2 \ x \ 10^3} \ kCal$

$= \frac{250}{4.2} \approx 60 \ kCal$

$2 \ Litres \ = \ 2000 \ cm^3$

Thus, each cm^3 of water is heated by $\frac{60 \ kCal}{2000} = -30°C$

$Final \ Temperature \ = \ initial \ temperature \ + \ change \ in \ temperature$

$= \ 25 \ + \ 30 \ = \ 55°C$

Question 17: E

E is the correct sequence. Remember sensory neurone take sensory information to the brain, and motor neurones take information away.

Question 18: F

The information given can only be used to work out the empirical formula. You would need to know the molar mass in order to calculate the chemical formula.

Question 19: A

Don't be afraid of how difficult this initially looks. If you follow the pattern, you get (e-e) which = 0. Anything multiplied by 0 gives zero.

Question 20: B

Intra-thoracic volume must decrease during expiration. Thus, the intercostal muscles relax causing the ribs must move down and in. The diaphragm moves up as well.

Question 21: F

$1 + (3\sqrt{2} - 1)^2 + (3 + \sqrt{2})^2$

$= 1 + (18 - 2(3\sqrt{2}) + 1) + (9 + 2(3\sqrt{2}) + 2)$

$= 31 - 6\sqrt{2} + 6\sqrt{2} = \underline{31}$

Question 22: B

The trick in this question is to conserve your units to prevent silly mistakes from creeping in. $200 \ cm^{-3} \ = \ 0.2 \ dm^{-3}$

$Number \ of \ moles \ = \ concentration \ x \ volume$ so: $0.2 \ x \ 1.8 \ = \ 0.36 \ mol$

Question 23: D
Using $s = ut + 0.5at^2$.
$125 = 0.5 \times 10 \times t^2$
$125 = 5 t^2$
$t = 5$ seconds
Therefore the final speed is $50ms^{-1}$, and the momentum is about $50ms^{-1} \times 0.4g = 20kgms^{-1}$.

Question 24: E
The most effective method in minimising side effects would be to only target bacteria. Only bacteria have a flagellum.

Question 25: E
Group 6 elements are non-metals whilst group 3 elements are metals. Thus, the group 3 element must lose electrons when it reacts with the group 6 element. The donation of electrons from its outer shell will decrease atomic size.

Question 26: D
It is extremely helpful to draw diagrams to simplify this.
Shaded area = area of circle – area of square
The area of the circle is $\pi r^2 = 3 \times 1^2 = 3cm^2$.
We don't know the side length of the square, but we do know the length of the diagonal is 2 cm, splitting the shape into two triangles.
The hypotenuse is therefore = radius x 2 = 2
Using Pythagoras' theorem, $2^2 = x^2 + x^2$ (where x = length and width of square)
Hence $2x^2 = 4$
$x^2 = 2$ = the area of the square
Therefore, the shaded area = $3 – 2 = 1cm^2$

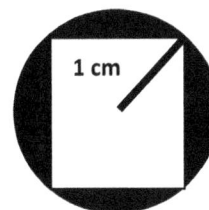

Question 27: B
The energy stored on descent is equal to the change in gravitational potential energy. The same energy is required to increase the height again, with an excess of the energy needed to lift the passengers. The energy needed to lift the passengers is therefore = $mg\Delta h = 72 \times 10 \times 10 \times 80 = 576kJ$. If the carriage moves at $4ms^{-1}$ for 200m, it takes 50 seconds to ascend. Therefore the rate of energy transfer is $576/50 = 11.52kJs^{-2} = 11.52kW$.

END OF SECTION

Section 3

'Doctors know best and should decide which treatment a patient receives'

Explain what this statement alludes to. Argue to the contrary that patients know best and should be able to choose their management plan. To what extent do you agree with this statement?

The statement describes paternalistic medicine in which it is assumed that since a doctor has been through years of training and experience, they are in the best place to consider the patients best interests and choose the most appropriate management plan. Patient autonomy is one of the core tenants of medicine. Since it is the patient's body, they should be fully informed about the range of treatments available, and their respective side effects, before deciding which treatment to receive.

There is already a power imbalance between doctors and patients, with patients often being in the most vulnerable stage of their lives. There is potential for this imbalance to be abused by some doctors – patients will often blindly follow whatever a doctor tells them simply because they are in the position of power. Paternalistic medicine further distorts this power balance towards doctors while patient autonomy helps the patient reclaim some power.

Even if all doctors are assumed to be benevolent, they are simply acting in the best interests of their patients, to the best of their knowledge. With a paternalistic approach, management is purely based on medical facts and a patient's lifestyle factors are not taken into account. This could have a large impact on the efficacy of management. E.g. Negative side effects leading to poor compliance.

Not only would the involvement of patients in treatment choices lead to better compliance (and therefore efficacy), involving patients in the decision making process may demystify a very complex and foreign topic and help ease any worries or concerns they have, leading to a more holistic, beneficial form of management.

I agree with the statement to the extent that doctors have been trained in medicine and are vastly experienced. However, I believe this experience would be best utilized by presenting the patient with the full range of treatment options in a manner they can understand, together with respective success rates/ side effects so that patients can make an informed decision as to which treatment they would like to receive. With this approach, patient autonomy is maintained, the patient would be able to consider which management plan is most compatible with their lifestyle and at the same time, the experience and knowledge of doctors would be provided at all times to help both parties to come to an informed decision together about the best overall management plan.

'World peace will be achieved in the future'

Explain what this statement means. Argue to the contrary, that world peace will never be achieved. To what extent, if any, do you agree with the statement?

This statement is ambiguous to define. It could mean no wars between nations, militaries and organisations or it could mean a world without murder or violence between humans. I would take world peace to mean an end to armed conflicts between nations and organisations but not necessarily a cessation of violence between individuals as this would be labelled as crime (as the scale of these acts cannot be considered a world problem or event).

Divisive issues will always arise between nations. There have been countless organisations (including the U.N., the league of nations and even the catholic church) that have attempted to bring nations to the negotiating table to work around these issues and to not rely on military force. However, despite their increasing power and influence over time, all have failed to prevent war.

Countries and organisation have spent vast sums of money purchasing arms and cumulative destructive ability has never been higher. Countries and organisations will always do this in order to ensure that their neighbours/rivals are not more powerful than them. To remove the enormous military capability that countries possess individual countries would need to be persuaded to disarm giving their rivals an advantage and removing the mutually assured destruction that underlies most of the stability in the modern day. Even if worldwide disarmament were achieved it would be difficult to maintain the world in this unstable state as rival countries or organisations could restart even minor arms races.

Man is intrinsically violent. Evolution has crafted man to identify any threats, whether from other species or other humans and to be able to react to these with force in order to survive. On the other hand there has been a steady drop in violence over the last few centuries which shows no sign of reversing in the future. This is true for both wars as well as crimes, it is easy to mislead by the raw data which is confounded by the huge increase in population over the last few hundred years but it is undoubtedly safer to be alive now than at any other time in history.
The world is becoming increasingly interconnected both in terms of economics and populations so wars have more impact now than ever. This provides a large disincentive for conflicts to arise that will only increase as human society integrates further.
As education increases the use of violence will no longer be accepted as a method conflict resolution.

Gains have been made in reducing conflict due to the interconnectivity of world trade and indeed its differing societies. Furthermore there are many powerful organisations that are designed to prevent conflict from taking place.
On the other hand these organisations have all failed to prevent wars. Furthermore disarming nations could actually lead to a decrease in stability as in provides an incentive for any nation to resist de-armament as doing so gives them a huge advantage over their rivals. Thus in conclusion I would argue that world peace is possible but unlikely.

'Medicine is a science; not an art'

Explain what this statement means. Argue to the contrary that medicine is in fact an art using examples to illustrate your answer. To what extent, if any, is medicine a science?

The statement suggests that medicine like science, is objective and quantifiable; a patient's symptoms and observations can be 'measured' to hypothesise a diagnosis which can then be treated empirically, in essence, evidence based medicine, rather than like an art, which is more subjective.

However, many would argue medicine is still an art. Patients don't behave like textbook examples, with the multiplicity of pathophysiological mechanisms meaning there are several different ways to arrive at the same disease, and the same disease manifesting in several different ways. This would be too complex to analyse using a simple measurement based approach and so a certain amount of intuition and creativity is needed when approaching patients.

Furthermore, pathophysiology is only half of medicine, with the actual interaction with the patient being as, if not more important. While there may be algorithms for communications skills, there is still no real science behind people skills and good bedside manner. To see how medicine could be considered an art, you simply have to watch a skilled physician communicate effortlessly with a patient.

Art can be used to describe any skill, which takes time and patience to master – many clinical skills easily fit into these criteria. The most extreme example that could be considered is a plastic surgeon, someone who is to all extents and purposes an artist with the human body as their canvass.

Despite this, I do still believe medicine is to a large extent still a science, and increasingly so. In every patient interaction, a clinician uses their underlying understanding of the first principles of science to come up with a hypothesis of a patients illness, which is then tested with further investigations before being managed empirically with evidence based medicine; the entire encounter is an illustration of the scientific process. Furthermore, management guidelines from NICE and other organisations are increasingly removing the intuitive aspect of management previously seen in medicine, and increasingly so as numerous studies continue to prove both efficacy and patient safety is improved with the use of guideline based medicine over intuitive medicine.

'People should live healthier lives to reduce the financial burden of healthcare to the taxpayer.'

Explain what this statement means. Argue to the contrary. To what extent do you agree with the statement?

The statement basically argues that by providing a financial encouragement to the individual to live healthy, the overall situation of public health will change. This is supposed to have a positive effect on the overall balance sheet of health care as financial encouragement is still cheaper than the treatment of disease. The thought is therefore that it is justified to pay money to reduce the occurrence of disease overall, at least in areas where disease can be prevented or reduced in incidence by mere healthy living. As statistically speaking this represents an increasingly great amount of overall burden on medical facilities, the argument does seem to have some validity.

There are some problems that arise from phrases like the one above. This lends itself well for counter arguments. One argument is the question, if it is acceptable to essentially influence the individual's free will and right to make their own decisions by providing them with an active encouragement to alter their behaviour. In a way this can be compared to training animals in the form that they receive a treat every time they do what their owner sees as positive and desirable. Another issue arises from the fact that only some diseases can be prevented by healthier life-style choices and that there is by no means a guarantee that healthy living will keep you free of disease.

Even if we ignore the counter arguments mentioned above, there are some issues with ideas such as these, the most obvious being the question of regulation. How can we monitor whether an individual is actually making healthy life-style choices and therefore is deserving of the promised bonus? Monitoring through medical tests will produce both, administrative as well as purely operative costs which will have to be taken into consideration when arguing that a bonus system will save money. Detailed monitoring of the individual's behaviour on the other hand is extremely difficult and most importantly raises the critical question of the individual's right of privacy from the government. Concerning the impact on the provision of healthcare, a financial bonus system might therefore reduce the overall cost of life-style associated diseases, but will cause a myriad of other costs and necessary medical processes that will make its effectiveness questionable.

All in all a financial bonus system seems like it might have a positive effect on the overall expenditure on healthcare, but upon closer inspection it becomes clear that the issue is a very complex one, this in turn makes its usefulness as a tool for the conservation of resources all the more questionable. Whilst it is a good idea to encourage the individual to life healthy and to do their best to avoid diseases that can be avoided, a system relying on financial encouragement might not be the right path to success.

END OF PAPER

MOCK PAPER F ANSWERS
Section 1

Question 1: D

Answer C) is completely irrelevant, so is not a flaw. Answer B) is not a flaw because when assessing an argument, anything that is stated (i.e. not concluded from other reasons in the passage) is accepted as true. We do not require evidence or sources for any statistics presented. Answers A) and E) are both claiming that something is immoral, which is thus expressing an opinion on the part of the arguer. This is not a flaw, the arguer is at liberty to claim something is immoral, and to claim that the government is morally obliged to act, and that it has not done so. Also, E) claims that *arguably* this is the most outrageous flaw of the government, clearly expressing an opinion, which is thus not required to be supported. However, answer D) identifies a valid flaw. The argument rests on us accepting that if there were less uninsured drivers, there would be less crashes. This is not necessarily correct, so D) is a flaw in the passage.

Question 2: A

The sentence 'Thus, the situation in Brazil is not applicable to the UK, and legalising gun ownership in the UK would be a bad move' gives the main conclusion of the argument and this is summarised in Answer A). Answer B) is partially supported by the passage, but the main conclusion concerns the situation in the UK and the passage states that there is little black market in the UK. Answer C) is incorrect as the passage only talks about gun ownership, not violent crime more generally. Answer D) is not fully supported by the passage, which states only that legalising guns would result in it being *easier* for criminals to acquire guns, not that there would be a large increase in their number. Answer E) is not the main conclusion as it focuses on an aspect of the evidence from Brazil, rather than the main conclusion which focuses on gun legislation in the UK.

Question 3:C

For each of the walls where there is no door, the wall is 6 tiles high and 5 tiles wide, which is 30 tiles. The wall where the door is requires a row of 2 tiles above the door, then there is a width of wall of 120cm which requires completely tiling, which is 6 tiles high and 3 tiles wide, hence this wall requires a total of 20 tiles. Hence a total of 110 tiles are required for the walls. The floor is 2 metres by 2 metres, so 5 tiles by 5 tiles, hence 25 tiles are required for the floor. Hence the answer is 135.

Question 4: D

Answer E) is irrelevant to which of Trevor and Jane will arrive first, so does not weaken the conclusion. Answers A), B) and C) all strengthen the answer, giving further reasons why we might expect Trevor to arrive first. Answer D), however, would slow Trevor down, meaning that it was more likely that Jane would arrive first. Thus, Answer D) weakens the passage's conclusion, and hence Answer D) is the answer.

Question 5: A

He has enough butter to make 2.5 times as many cupcakes as the recipe, which is 50
He has enough sugar to make 3 times as many cupcakes as the recipe, which is 60
He has enough flour to make 5 times as many cupcakes as the recipe, which is 100
He has enough eggs to make 34 times as many cupcakes as the recipe, which is 60
The lowest of these is 50, so he makes 50 cupcakes. He needs 2.5 x 4 eggs to do this, which is 10 eggs. Therefore he has 2 eggs left over.

Question 6: B

Let the number of minutes the journey takes be t. Therefore, ABC charge 400+15t pence for the journey. We can calculate that XYZ taxis charge 400+(30x6) pence, = 580 pence. Therefore, for both journeys to cost the same, 580=400+15t. 180=15t, therefore t=12. Therefore the 6 mile journey needs to take 12 minutes. 6 miles in 12 minutes is 30 miles per hour, so the answer is B.

Question 7: E

We can see that all of answers A) through D) are essential for the conclusion to be valid from the squire's reasoning. Lancelot must have great courage, this must be a requirement for the Adzol, and no other knights must have sufficient courage, in order for us to be certain that Lancelot will succeed but all of Arthur's other knights will fail. Thus A) and B) can be clearly identified as assumptions. C) and D) require a bit more thought, but we can see that nothing in the passage explicitly states the Elders' tales are correct. If the elders are not correct, then great courage may not be required to be successful in the Adzol. Thus, both C) and D) are also assumptions. Hence, the answer is E).

Question 8: E

B) is incorrect, as the passage does not say that arch-shaped gaps *always* indicate where windows once stood, simply that *these arches* do. C) is also incorrect, as the passage simply states that windows are not found in *underground halls*. A) is a reason in the passage, and is not a conclusion. D) and E) could both be described as conclusions from this passage, but we see that if we accept D) as true (along with the fact that the hall is now underground), we have good reason to believe that E) is true, whereas E) being true does not necessarily mean that D) is true. Thus, E) is the *main* conclusion, whilst D) is an *intermediate conclusion*, which supports the main conclusion.

Question 9: D

Usually bread rolls cost 30p for a pack, but if the cost per bread roll is reduced by 1p then they will cost 24p. Hence we need to find z, where $24(z+1)=30z$, where z is the original number of packs that could have been afforded. $24z+24=30z$, hence $24=6z$, so $z=4$. Hence he was originally supposed to be buying 4 packets of bread rolls, which is $6 \times 4 = 24$ rolls.

Question 10: B

Answer E) is an irrelevant statement that says nothing about whether England *do* have good players. Answers A) and D) actually weaken the sporting director's arguments, suggesting that England may have a good team, and it may just be poor performances in world cups, and not a lack of talented players. This leaves B) and C). C) may appear to strengthen the sporting director's argument, but on closer inspection we see that in fact it says that for the last 70 years, England have had at least 1 player in the top 10 in the world. This does *not* strengthen the argument that England have been lacking talent for the last 25 years, and may actually reinforce the chairman's argument that it is simply the *current* crop of players that are not good enough. Answer B), however, does strengthen the argument, suggesting that England's performances have been poor over the last 20 years, thus strengthening the argument that there may be a lack of talented players that has been ongoing for a couple of decades, as claimed by the sporting director.

Question 11: A

He can prepare each batch of cakes while the previous one is in the oven but it takes longer so we have to allow 25 minutes for each batch, plus 20 minutes for the last batch to cook while no further batch is being prepared. There are 12 in each batch, so for 100 cupcakes there needs to be 9 batches. Hence the total time needed is 25 minutes x 9, + 20 minutes. This is 245 minutes, or 4 hours 5 minutes. Hence to be ready by 4pm he needs to start at 11:55am, so the answer is A.

Question 12: D

We can first work out the rate of girls' absenteeism. First we need to work out how many of the pupils at Heather Park Academy and Holland Wood Comprehensive are girls. Let g be the number of girls in Heather Park Academy. Then $0.06(g)+0.05(1000-g)=(1000)(0.056)$. Then $0.06g-0.05g=56-50$. Then $0.01g=6$, so $g = 600$. Hence 600 pupils at Heather Park Academy are girls. The proportions at Holland Wood Comprehensive are the same but there are half as many pupils, so 900 pupils at the two schools combined are girls.

The average absenteeism of girls is 7%. We know that 900 of the 1100 girls have an average absenteeism rate of 6%. Let the average absenteeism rate of girls at Hurlington Academy be r. Then $900 \times 0.06 +200r = 0.07 \times 1100$. Hence $54+200r=77$. $77-54 = 200r$. $23/200 = r$. $r=0.115$. Hence, the rate of absenteeism amongst girls at Hurlington Academy is 11.5%

Question 13: C

A), B) D) and E) are all directly stated in the passage, so can all be reliably concluded. Perhaps the trickiest of these to see is answer D), which is true because the passage says "*due to*" the advent of more accurate technology, thus clearly identifying that this had *caused* the switch to the situation of most watches being made by machine. C), however, is *not* necessarily true. The passage states that most *watches* are produced by machines, but only states that *some* watchmakers now only perform repairs. This does not necessarily mean that most watchmakers do not produce watches. It could be that only a handful are required in the entirety of the watch industry for repairs, and that the numbers still producing watches exceeds those in the repair business. Thus, C) cannot be reliably concluded from the passage.

Question 14: A

B) is not a valid conclusion from the passage, because the fact that someone uses an illogical argument (as some pescatarians are claimed to in this passage) does not mean that they cannot use logic. D) and E) are not conclusions from this passage because the passage is not saying anything about the ethicality of eating meat, but simply commenting that one argument used against doing so is not logical. Answers C) and A) are both valid conclusions from the passage, but we see that if we accept C) as being true, it gives us good cause to believe that A) is true, but this does not apply the other way round. Thus, C) is an intermediation conclusion, whilst A) is the main conclusion.

Question 15: E

The research conducted does not ask about whether it is *important* to learn some of the language before travelling abroad, simply whether participants *would*, so B) cannot be concluded. D) is incorrect because the passage states *15%* would, which is clearly not less than 10%. The passage states that this is symptomatic of a deeper underlying issue, but does not say that many issues of racism stem from this, so C) cannot be concluded. Now, the passage states that 60% of people feel foreign people should learn English before travelling to Britain, and 15% of people would attempt to learn the language before travelling to a country which did not speak English. However, this 15% could be some of the same people as the 60%, in which case A) would be incorrect. Thus, A) cannot be reliably concluded. However, there must be at least 45% of people who feel that foreign people should learn English, but would not learn a foreign language themselves, so E) *can* be reliably concluded.

Question 16: D

She needs to print 400 x 2 = 800 double sided A4 sheets, which will cost 0.01 x 2 x 1.5 = £0.03 each. Hence the total cost of this is 800 x 0.03 = £24. She also needs to print 1500 single sided A5 sheets, costing £0.01 each, giving a total of 1500 x 0.01 = £15. Hence the total cost is £39.

Question 17: B

The passage has stated that if Kirkleatham win the game they will win the league, so E) is not an assumption. Meanwhile, the manager has stated A), C) and D), and the passage has not claimed anything about whether Kirkleatham can easily win the game, so A) and D) are not assumptions. However, B) does identify an assumption in the passage. The fact that Kirkleatham will not win the game without playing with desire and commitment does *not* mean that they will win the game if they do play with desire and commitment. And we can see that for the argument's conclusion (that Kirkleatham *will* definitely win the league) to be valid from its reasoning, this is required to be true. Thus, B) identifies an assumption in the passage.

Question 18: B

Answers A) and E) are not relevant, because neither affect the strength of the councillor's argument from a critical thinking point of view. The councillor's argument says nothing about house prices, simply the cost of building the estate and the effects on wildlife, so A) is not relevant. E) is not relevant because additional support, or likelihood that it will be heeded, does nothing to affect the strength of a given argument. C) and D) actually strengthen the councillor's argument, suggesting that brownfield land does have good infrastructure (C)) and that the greenbelt areas do have a lot of wildlife (D)). B) does weaken the councillor's argument, as it suggests that building on brownfield land may also have adverse impacts on wildlife.

Question 19: A

England won Pool C so they will be in Quarterfinal 3, where they will play Brazil. If they win, they will play the winner of Quarterfinal 1. Hence they can only meet teams from Quarterfinals 2 or 4 in the final. These teams are Argentina, Nigeria, South Africa or Holland. Hence the only one of these 5 teams they can play in the final is Nigeria.

Question 20: B

We can tell the amounts for the green party and the blue party are both 1/3 of the total, and that the amount for the red party is 1/4 of the total. Hence 1/12 is left, so the amount for the yellow party must be 1/12. Hence the red party have 3 times the intended vote of the yellow party.

Question 21: B

A large pizza wish mushrooms and ham is £12, garlic bread is £3, chips are £1.50 x 2 = £3, a dip is £1, hence the current total is £19. The cheapest way to order this is to get the price up to exactly £30 as this will reduce the price to £18. This takes £11. Only one of these options costs £11, which is a large pizza with mushroom. Hence the answer is B.

Question 22: E

In Rovers' first 3 games, they have scored 1 goal and had 8 goals scored against them. In total they scored 1 goal and had 10 goals scored against them, so they must have lost their last game against United 2-0.
In City's first 3 games, they scored 7 goals and had 3 goals scored against them. In total they scored 10 goals and had 4 goals scored against them. Hence they must have won their game against United 3-1. Hence the answer is E.

Question 23: D

The question simply describes how a combination of factors are responsible for the M1 being the world's most formidable tank, so the view of country X is incorrect. It does *not* claim that it is impossible for a tank to be as good as the M1 Abrams, so E) is not a valid conclusion. Equally, it does not say the new tank's armour will not be as good as the Abrams (in fact it is implied that it may well be as good), so C) is also incorrect. A) B) and D) are all valid conclusions from this passage, but we can see that A) and B) contribute towards supporting the conclusion in D). Thus, D) is the main conclusion of this passage, whereas A) and B) are *intermediate* conclusions given to support this main conclusion.

Question 24: D

We can simply add up the amounts in the bank accounts and find the difference between each month – it doesn't matter that the salary is paid in as it is the same every month. Doing this, we find out the biggest difference is between 1st May and 1st June, hence the answer is D, May.

Question 25 : B

Firstly we can work out the full dose for the son. He needs to take 0.2ml per kg of weight for each dose, and he is 40kg, so this is 8ml. He takes 40 doses altogether, so in total he needs 320ml of medicine.
Then we work out the doses for everyone else, add them together and half them. The daughter's full dose would be 2ml, 30 times, which is 60ml altogether. My dose would be 7.5ml, 60 times, which is 450ml. My husband's dose would be 8ml, 60 times, which is 480ml. Altogether, this is 990ml. However, only half of these dosages is needed, which is 495ml. Hence the total needed is 320 + 495, which is 815ml. Hence 5 200ml bottles of medicine are needed for the full course.

Question 26: A

There are 21 forks and 21 knives. If half as many are red as blue, and half as many are blue as yellow, they are in the ratio red:blue:yellow 1:2:4. Hence of the 21, 3 are red, 6 are blue and 12 are yellow. Hence the probability of getting a yellow knife is 12/21 = 4/7. The probability of getting a red fork is 3/21 = 1/7. Hence the probability of getting both is (1/7) x (4/7) = 4/49.

Question 27: D

The Principle used in the passage is that public funds raised through taxation (which is compulsory) should not be used for any services unless they benefit everyone, such that nobody is forced to pay for services that do not benefit them. Answer D) is the best application of this principle, as it directly follows it. Answer B) mentions public funds being used to support a service that benefits the whole country, but this does not necessarily mean that they *shouldn't* be used to support services that don't benefit everyone, so answer B) is not as directly an application of the principle as answer D). Answer E) is not the same principle because this is talking about funds being used for services that benefit the *country*, rather than everyone in it. Meanwhile, Answer A) is talking about how many people *use* a certain service, rather than how many people *benefit* from it, so this is not the same principle. Answer C) is completely different talking about funds being used because some cannot afford private health service, regardless of how many people are benefitting from the public health service.

Question 28: B

The chairman has *stated* that All inclusive services are more popular than Hourly services. He has not deduced this from any evidence, and thus he has assumed nothing about their popularity. Thus, C) and D) are incorrect. The chairman's argument is simply that focusing on All inclusive services will bring in more profit than Hourly services, as he says they should focus on All inclusive *rather* than Hourly services. Thus, any reference to other services or other profit-raising strategies are irrelevant, so A) and E) are irrelevant. However, B) correctly identifies the chairman's flaw. Just because All inclusive is more *popular* than Hourly services does not mean they are more *profitable*, and if they are not then the chairman's conclusion is no longer valid. Thus, B) correctly identifies the flaw in his argument.

Question 29: A

B) is not an assumption because the passage *states* that renewable sources do not cause damage, so we accept this as true. E) is not a flaw, because again the passage has stated that the use of these fuels to produce power will continue to cause climate change *as long as it continues*, thus we must accept as true that it cannot be halted or prevented whilst these fuels are used. C) and D) are irrelevant to the argument's conclusion that if we wish to stop damage to the environment, we need to switch to renewable fuels, and thus they are not flaws. However, at no point is it stated that *all* non-renewable fuel sources cause environmental damage, it is only stated the non-renewables *such as* oil, coal and natural gas do. Thus, we have no guarantee that Nuclear fuel will cause environmental damage, and if it doesn't, the passage's conclusion no longer stands. Thus, A) is a valid assumption in the passage.

Question 30: E

Answers A) and D) do *not* strengthen or weaken the argument because the question states that this increase in non-vaccinated individuals has occurred despite powerful evidence of vaccine safety, and in spite of advice from doctors. This suggests that people who do not vaccinate pay little attention to evidence of advice from doctors, so we should not expect these factors to have much of an effect. B) is completely irrelevant to whether the rate of increase will continue. C) actually weakens the argument, suggesting that such increases are common, and normally stop after 6 years. If the current increase was to follow suit, it would stop next year and vaccination rates would not fall below 90%. E), however, implies that this kind of increase has happened only once before, and in this case it continued for 13 years. If the current increase was to follow *this* pattern, it would continue for another 8 years, where vaccination rates would be below 90%. Thus, E) strengthens the argument's conclusion that we should expect an outbreak of measles.

Question 31: C

The percentage of students who had their grades predicted correctly is the same as the number who had their grades predicted correctly as there are 100. Hence we simply need to add up the numbers on the diagonal of the table, where actual grade is the same as predicted. This adds up to 39, hence the answer is C.

Question 32: B

The 2 wage reductions mean that when the wage increases happen, the raises will be x% of a smaller number than the decreases were. Thus, the wage will not rise as high as the original level.

If you are struggling to visualise this, the easiest way to do it is to substitute a number for x. Let us do the calculation treating x as 10. The first wage drop is by 10%. Thus, the wage is now 90% of the original wage.

The second wage drop is also by 10%, but at this point, the wage is only 90% of the original wage. Thus, the drop will be by 10% *of 90%* of the original wage, resulting in a new wage of 81% of the original wage (10% of 90% is 9%)

Then, we have the first increase, which will be 10% of this new wage (81% of the original wage). Thus, after the first increase, the new wage will be 81% +(10% of 81%) of the original wage. Thus, it will be 81% + 8.1%, which is 89.1% of the original wage.

Now we have the second increase. Another 10% is added, this time of 89.1% of the original wage. We now have an increase of 8.91% (10% of 89.1). Thus, after the final raise, the wage will be 89.1% + 8.91%, which is 98.01% of the original wage. Thus, the new wage is lower than the original wage.

END OF SECTION

Section 2

Question 1: G

The replacement of dying, damaged, and lost cells, the growth of the embryonic cell to a multi-cellular organism, and asexual reproduction are the three main reasons why cells divide through mitosis.

Question 2; F

This question will discriminate between students who spot short-cuts built into questions to save valuable time and those that simply dive straight in without appraising the question.

The key here is that due to the conservation of energy, all the gravitational potential energy, mgh, at the top of the ramp will be converted to kinetic energy, ½mv², at the bottom.

Thus, we can calculate the final velocity using the following: mgh = ½mv²

Note that the mass cancels so there is no need to use the density and volume information in order to calculate mass.

Hence we get: 2gh = v²

V² = 2 x 10 x 20 = 400

Therefore, v = 20 ms⁻¹

Question 3: C

Transition metals form multiple stable ions which may have many different colours (e.g. green Fe_{2+} and brown Fe_{3+}). They usually form ionic bonds and are commonly used as catalysts (e.g. iron in the Haber process, Nickel in alkene hydrogenation). They are excellent conductors of electricity and are known as the d-block elements.

Question 4: D

Waves do not transfer mass, but their net neutral motions can interfere with each other to cause standing waves or other interference patterns. The energy of a wave depends on frequency, so waves have many different energies. Gamma rays have the highest energy for light, while visible light is lower in energy.

Question 5: C

A sensory receptor (1) senses the heat of the pan. This information is passed down the sensory neurone (2) through a relay neurone to the motor neurone (4), which then causes the muscle (5) to contract, pulling the finger away.

Question 6: C

The receptor is directly coupled to the sensory neurone, so the communication here is electrical. All information between neurones passes via synapses, which use neurotransmitters to convey the information chemically. This occurs between the sensory neurone and the relay neurone, and between the relay neurone and the motor neurone. Therefore, the answer is C).

Question 7: A

This is an example of an addition reaction: the chloride and hydrogen atoms are added at the unsaturated bond of the but-2-ene, which is between the 2ⁿᵈ and the 3ʳᵈ C-atom. If you're unsure about this type of question draw it out and the answer will be obvious.

Question 8: A

Multiply by the denominator to give: $(7x + 10) = (3z^2 + 2)(9x + 5)$

Partially expand brackets on right side: $(7x + 10) = 9x(3z^2 + 2) + 5(3z^2 + 2)$

Take x terms across to left side: $7x - 9x(3z^2 + 2) = 5(3z^2 + 2) - 10$

Take x outside the brackets: $x[7 - 9(3z^2 + 2)] = 5(3z^2 + 2) - 10$

Thus: $x = \frac{5(3z^2+2)-10}{7-9(3z^2+2)}$

Simplify to give: $x = \frac{(15z^2)}{[7 - 9(3z^2 + 2)]}$

Question 9: C

The electrolysis reaction for brine is: $2\ NaCl\ +\ 2\ H_2O\ =\ 2\ NaOH\ +\ H_2\ +\ Cl_2$

Thus, keeping in mind the stoichiometry of the given equation, the solution must be C.

Question 10: B

An alpha particle is a helium nucleus consisting of 2 protons and 2 neutrons. An alpha decay therefore reduces the atomic (proton) number by 2 and the mass number by 4. After a single alpha decay, the resulting proton number is 88 and the resulting mass number is 184. As this then splits in to two, the resulting element has a proton number of 44 and a mass number of 92. Gamma radiation does not alter the subatomic particle make-up of an atom.

Question 11: A

If the two isotopes were in equal abundance, the A_r would be 77, half-way between the two isotope masses (the average). The A_r is 76.5 (a weighted average), one quarter of the way between the isotopes, so there must be three times as much of the lighter isotope to move the A_r closer to its mass of 76 (0.75x76 + 0.25x78 = 76.5).

Though there is more of ^{76}X than ^{78}X, this does not necessarily imply that ^{78}X is lost through decay, as opposed to naturally less abundant from the beginning, so there is no way to know the relative stability of the isotopes.

Question 12: C

Increasing the concentration of the reactants (not products) would affect reaction rate, which can be monitored by measuring the gas volume released (proportional to molar concentration). This is the reaction for photosynthesis, which does not occur spontaneously and is endothermic.

Question 13: H

Most polymers are made up of alkenes, which are unsaturated molecules. Polymerisation does not release water, as it is an addition reaction. Depending on the monomer molecule, polymers can take a variety of shapes.

Question 14: B

The shortest distance between points A and B is a direct line. Using Pythagoras:

The diagonal of a sports field $= \sqrt{40^2 + 30^2} = \sqrt{1,600 + 900} = \sqrt{2,500} = 50$.

The diagonal between the sports fields $= \sqrt{4^2 + 3^2} = \sqrt{16 + 9} = \sqrt{25} = 5$.

Thus, the shortest distance between A and B $= 50 + 5 + 50 = 105\ m$.

Question 15: C

Let $y = 1.25$ x 10^8; this is not necessary, but helpful, as the question can then be expressed as: $\frac{100y + 10y}{2y} = \frac{110y}{2y} = 55$

Question 16: D

Taking the diseased allele to be X^D and X as the normal allele, we can model the scenario in the Punnett square below:

		Carrier Mother	
		X^D	X
Diseased Father	X^D	X^DX^D	X^DX
	Y	X^DY	XY

Boys are XY and girls are XX. 50% of the boys produced would have DMD. So the probability that both boys would have the disease is 0.5 x 0.5 = 0.25

Question 17: E

We can see from the Punnett square that the probability of having a girl with DMD is 25% (X^DX^D). The probability that both are girls with DMD is 0.25 x 0.25 = 0.125.

Question 18: C
Chemical reactions take place in the cytoplasm, and the mitochondrion is the site for aerobic respiration releasing energy. The lack of a cell wall means that this is an animal cell.

Question 19: A
Equate y to give:
$2x - 1 = x^2 - 1$
$\rightarrow x^2 - 2x = 0$
$\rightarrow x(x - 2) = 0$
Thus, x = 2 and x = 0
There is no need to substitute back to get the y values as only option A satisfies the x values.

Question 20: B
The ruler and the cruise ship look to be the same size because their edges are in line with Tim's line of sight. His eyes form the apex of two similar triangles. All the sides of two similar triangles are in the same ratio since the angles are the same, therefore:

$$\frac{0.3\,m}{X\,m} = \frac{1\,m}{1\,m + 999\,m}$$

Thus, $X\,m = 1000\,m \times \frac{0.3\,m}{1\,m}$

$1000 \times 0.3 = 300\,m$

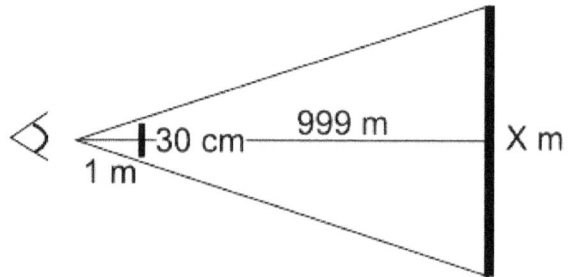

Question 21: A
As energy is added to ice, the molecules increase their vibrations and the temperature increases. As the ice begins to melt, all energy goes into breaking the bonds to form water, and none goes to increasing the temperature. Once all bonds are broken, the energy again goes to increasing the temperature of the water.

Question 22: D
White blood cells can engulf/phagocytose pathogens in order to kill them. CO_2 is transported in the plasma, not in blood cells.

Question 23: B
The Doppler Effect applies to all waves including members of the electromagnetic spectrum. A wave emitted from a moving object, like the sound from a siren, will be compressed as it moves toward you, causing sounds or light of higher frequency (pitch, energy). When an ambulance drives toward you, the siren will become higher in pitch, as it drives past it will move neither towards or away from you, so there will be no Doppler Effect, then the Doppler Effect will cause a lower pitch as it drives away and the waves are stretched to longer wavelengths.

Question 24: C
Power= Current x Voltage
Thus, one battery generates: 1.2 V x 2500 mAh
= 1.2 V x 2.5 Ah = 3 Watt hours

The light uses: 30 W x 1 h = 30 Wh

Therefore, it will take 30 Wh / 3 Wh = 10 batteries to power the light for one hour.

Question 25: C
Electric conduction is a consequence of metallic bonding: metal atoms lose their valence electrons to obtain their optimum energy state, with the cations forming a lattice held together by electromagnetic attraction to the cloud of free electrons. These free electrons can then conduct electricity, as they are not bound to any particular atom. This does not require the movement of ions or the breaking of the cation lattice.

Question 26: D
The distance travelled is the area under the curve (v x t = d at every v and t, sum for each t to find the total d, which also is the area; think of the case for constant v if confused).
Each square corresponds to 1 m (1 m/s x 1 s = 1 m), so counting squares gives an approximate distance of 30 m travelled: 31 m in a positive direction and 1 m in the negative direction (negative velocity).

Question 27: C
Let Bob = B, Kerry = K and Son = S.

$B = 2K, K = 3S$ and $B + K + S = 50$

$50 = 2K + K + \frac{K}{3} = \frac{6K}{3} + \frac{3K}{3} + \frac{K}{3}$
$50 = \frac{10K}{3}$

Hence: $10K = 150$

$K = 15$
$B = 2 \times 15 = 30$
$S = \frac{15}{3} = 5$

So: Bob's age when his son was born = 30 – 5 = 25.

END OF SECTION

Section 3

'A doctor should never disclose medical information about his patients'

What does this statement mean? Argue to the contrary using examples to strengthen your response. To what extent do you agree with this statement?

This statement addresses the issue of patient confidentiality, saying that there are no circumstance in which a doctor should reveal information about a patient's health to a third-party (be it friends, family, or stranger) without the patients informed knowledge and consent. For the purpose of this essay, I will assume that this excludes other medical staff who may also be involved in the patients care and argue that there are several situations in which it is valid to disclose patient information.

An important distinction has to be made between instances in which a doctor is legally required to disclose medical information and instances when a doctor may choose to disclose medical information about a patient.

There are several instances in which it is legally required for doctors to disclose patient information, regardless of patient consent. For example, there is a list of notifiable diseases including meningitis and tuberculosis that have to be reported in the interest of infection control and patient safety. Other legal requirements include information about road traffic accidents, potential terrorist activities, and coroner requests or in the court of law.

There are also other instances in which a doctor may be legally permitted to disclose information but need not necessarily do so. These tend to have their own host of ethical challenges and ultimately reside in the discretion of the doctor. For example, if a doctor suspects that a patient may have mental health issues or has mentioned something suggesting they may harm themselves or others, a doctor is legally permitted to bring it up with the relevant authorities, if they feel it is relevant. Another example may be cases in which a doctor suspects potential child abuse, and the doctor may choose to bring this up further with the authorities without the parents consent.

To a large extent, I do agree with the statement as patient confidentiality is one of the core tenants of medicine; patients place a huge amount of trust in doctors during one of the most vulnerable points of their life and this responsibility needs to be respected. However, as highlighted above, there are several cases in which a doctor is legally required/ permitted to disclose information about patients, and these tend to be in cases where disclosure results in greater good overall (to either the patient or the public) than patient confidentiality.

'Science is nothing more than just a thought process'

Explain what this statement means. Argue to the contrary, that science is much more than just a thought process. To what extent, if any, do you agree with the statement?

Science is obviously driven by the interpretation of information and the subsequent generation of hypothesis, this is what is referred to by the thought process in the title. *A precise definition of the meaning of the question is essential in directing subsequent discussion.*

However these observations are built on experimentation and observation that do not always require a specific thought process behind them. *Signpost the topics you are going to raise later.*

In addition to this we must consider that if something is discovered unintentionally is it still a scientific discovery. Is it important that the discovery advances Science or that it is made in a scientific manner.

Some aspects of science can be performed completely in the mind, mathematics and theoretical physics rely on insight generated by thinking and applying core axioms on which they are founded. *What is there in support of the statement, don't back away from offering strong arguments as they will be of value when coming to a conclusion.*

The scientific method is the generation and testing of hypothesis with the intention of proving them to be false, this is the basis of all science and it is very clearly a thought process, all of the experimentation done is directed by this.

There is a need for investigation in some areas where we have little knowledge and what would ideally be a spearhead of inquiry is often a broad net of hope. A good example of this is Genome Wide Association Studies (GWAS), these look for associations between gene variants and disease yet despite this there is no thought process behind this deeper than the need to generate information and provide new target genes for research.

In the same manner high throughput screening of chemical compounds to assess their function as potential pharmaceutical agents has no specified aim on undertaking. Any success that comes from such a process cannot be entirely attributed to the thought process, there is a large degree of serendipity.

Science in its purest form is a thought process but in reality it cannot be. There is a requirement for information to be generated so insight can be found. In many cases we must proceed without an expectation of the insight we will gain because without committing to an investigation we would not be able to have insight. This thought process is different from that stated in the title as it does not require a precise interpretation only a general line of inquiry.

In conclusion science is a thought process imposed on experimentation and observation, without the other each has no individual utility but information must be generated before it can be interpreted.

'With an ageing population, it's necessary to increase the individual's contribution to the healthcare system in order to maintain standards.'

Explain what this statement means. Argue to the contrary. To what extent do you agree with the statement?

Due to generally decreasing numbers of births and a constantly increasing longevity, our population grows increasingly old. As people live longer and there are less people born, the percentage of elderly individuals in the population grows in relation to the percentage of younger individuals that work and finance health care through their taxes. With increasing age, medical needs of the individual increase as well. Statistically speaking, the biggest need for medical attention and therefore the biggest consumption of healthcare assets happens in the last third of the individual's life. In order to maintain the current standard of support of the increasing amounts of elderly, it becomes necessary to spend more money on healthcare which in turn makes higher contributions of the individual necessary. It is important to recognise that when the NHS was established in 1948 the structure of society as a whole was a completely different one compared to what it is today.

There are several issues that arise from this statement that lend themselves well for counterarguments. One of the issues is the general structure of our healthcare system. This does not aim at the idea of free health care for all, but more at the idea of individual processes being unnecessarily complicated and inefficient consuming disproportional amounts of resources. Streamlining the structure of the NHS as well as the procedures in place can provide means of reducing overall expenditure. One other valid counterargument lies in the principle idea of the NHS to put an end to health care inequalities based on the individuals income. By increasing the individual contribution without adjustment of wages etc, a disproportionally heavy burden is placed on the less well of in comparison to the rich which essentially re-instates healthcare inequality on the basis of income.

There is this general idea of a responsibility between generations. Our parents and grandparents worked their whole life building the society we live in today. In a way we harvest the fruits of their labour today and for this reason it is our responsibility to care for the generations that came before us. It is therefore our duty to care for them to the best of our abilities. Issues such as the ones our healthcare system is facing today, make it increasingly difficult to fulfil this responsibility, especially with chronic morbidity becoming increasingly common, even in younger generations with diseases such as diabetes and metabolic syndrome affecting increasingly individuals in the second third of their life. Due to this increase in overall workload for the healthcare system, it seems unavoidable that the individuals contribution must be increased in order to maintain the same standard of care delivered today, unless the disease patterns of the population change.

'Assisted suicide allows those suffering from incurable diseases to die with dignity and without unnecessary pain.'

Explain what this statement means. Argue the contrary. To what extent do you agree with the statement?

The idea of euthanasia as a tool for pain control and palliative care is nothing new. Over the past years it has been raised over and over again in order to legalize the practice as is the case in some other countries such as the Switzerland. The argument behind the idea is that every individual has the right to decide what is to be done with their body and their life independent of what others might think provided that he or she is in control of their mental powers and are free of undue external influence. The idea of euthanasia as a possible form of treatment revolves around the concept that a medical professional has to accept the individuals decision for whatever form of treatment, even if this decision is considered unwise or might even lead to the individuals death. An additional component arises from the idea of dignity in general and in particular of dying in dignity. Everybody has a deep desire to be comfortable at the time of their death and the prospect of unbearable pain or complete loss of self is a wide-spread fear.

Some of the strongest arguments opposing euthanasia are philosophical ones. It evolves around the idea of how far human beings have the right to take another humans life. In addition to that euthanasia goes against everything that the medical profession stands for. The cure of disease and the saving of life and good health. Death will never cure a disease nor will it ever maintain life or good health. Other opposing arguments include the idea of actual consent to commit suicide. What happens with patients that are not able to communicate with the doctors or to what extend is it a possibility that relatives are 'talked into' feeling as a burden and wanting to end their lives for that reason. A final concern arises from the idea that allowing euthanasia for terminally ill patients or as a form of pain control will open the door to other arguments arguing for life in some cases not being worth living.

The idea of euthanasia may have a place in the theoretical realms of arguing medical care and the treatment of terminally ill patients. In real practice however it has little place. Whilst it can be argued that in some cases an individual might be happier dead rather than being alive, the dangers and concerns arising from the concept of euthanasia seem to outweigh these concerns and ultimately euthanasia goes against the very core ideas that form the basis of the medical profession.

END OF PAPER

MOCK PAPER G ANSWERS

Section 1

Question 1: C

Answer B) is completely irrelevant to what the manager is saying, so is incorrect. A) and E) are also incorrect as the manager is simply talking about ticket sales. He has not mentioned anything about the relevant popularity of folk music, or how much the band should value profit. D) is incorrect as the manager is simply saying that the band will have higher ticket sales in France than in Germany, so other countries are not relevant.

C) is correct as Germany could still have higher ticket sales for folk music than France despite the recent changes in ticket sales.

Question 2: D

Let the number of invitations with the extra information in be m. Invitations with extra information in cost £0.70 to send and invitations without cost £0.60. Therefore the total cost of posting is £0.70m + £0.60(50-m) and this is equal to £33. 33=0.70m-0.60m+30. 3=0.1m therefore m=30. So the number of invitations with extra information in is 30. Therefore the answer is D.

Question 3: B

Only B) is not an assumption, as it is stated in the question that both Grace and Rose departed at 5:15. The other answers are all assumptions. At no point has it been stated that both the girls are walking, or that they will walk at the same speed. If either of these points are incorrect, we cannot definitely state that they will arrive home at the same time. Therefore A) and E) are assumptions. Also, it has not been stated that the gymnastics class is being held at the local gymnasium. If this is not the case, then we cannot know how far Grace and Rose have to walk, and therefore cannot state that they will arrive home at the same time. Therefore, C) is an assumption. Equally, if Grace gets lost, she may arrive home after Rose, so D) is an assumption.

Question 4: E

Answer A) is completely irrelevant to John's conclusions, as the speed of travel has no effect on the train's destination. D) is also irrelevant as other destinations from King's Cross station also bear no effect on John's conclusion. Meanwhile, B) is incorrect as John's conclusions refer to travelling to Edinburgh by train, so the possibility of travelling by aeroplane has no effect. C) is not an assumption because John's conclusion is in the present tense, referring to journeys made at the moment, so future developments have no effect.

E) is an assumption John has made. Only two other stations in London have been mentioned. At no point has it been mentioned that there are no other stations in London that John could travel from.

Question 5: C

The question says that Shaniqua plays in the square which will stop Summer being able to win straight away, so Shaniqua must play in 4. Summer then needs to play in a square where there will be 2 different options to make a line on the turn afterwards, so that Shaniqua cannot block both of them. If Summer plays in 1, she can make a line by playing in either 5 or 6 the next turn, so Shaniqua cannot stop her winning. If Summer plays in 2, she cannot make a line on the next turn at all. If Summer plays in 3, she can only make a line by playing in 6 the next turn and so Shaniqua can stop her. If Summer plays in 5, she can only make a line by playing in 5 the next turn and so Shaniqua can stop her. If Summer plays in 6, she can make a line by playing in either 1 or 3 the next turn, so Shaniqua cannot stop her winning. Therefore she either needs to play in 1 or 6 to be able to be certain of winning the next time.

Question 6: C

B) and D) are both stated in the question. A) is also stated as the question states that Tanks were a hugely influential factor in ALL battles in World War 2.

E) is not stated but is not an assumption as it is not required to be true for the argument's conclusion to be valid.

C) However, is required to be true for the conclusion to be valid and yet is never stated in the question, so it is an assumption.

Question 7: B

D) is irrelevant to the argument's conclusion, whilst A) and E) are also irrelevant as the argument does not directly imply either of these things (and even if it did they are irrelevant to the argument's conclusions so are not flaws). C) is incorrect because the argument states that the Prussian arrival was essential to the British victory, so C) is not an assumption.

B), however, is never stated in the question, but is needed to be true for the argument's conclusion to be valid.

Question 8: B

D) and E) are both entirely irrelevant to waiting times, so are not flaws.

C) is not correct, as the question states that busier ports have longer queuing times. A) is also incorrect as the question states that Bordeux is the busiest port in France, so Calais is definitely less busy than Bordeux. Therefore, Porto cannot be busier than Bordeux but less busy than Calais.

B) is a flaw, as the fact that Bilbao was busiest last year does not necessarily mean it will be busy this year.

Question 9: B

The volume of the box with 10cm squares cut out is $10*100*100 = 100000cm^3$
The volume of the box with 20cm squares cut out is $20*80*80 = 128000cm^3$
The volume of the box with 30cm squares cut out is $30*60*60 = 108000cm^3$
The volume of the box with 40cm squares cut out is $40*40*40 = 64000cm^3$
The volume of the box with 50cm squares cut out is $50*20*20 = 20000cm^3$
Therefore the biggest box is the one with the 20cm squares cut out, so the answer is B.

Question 10: A

At no point is A) stated, but if aeroplanes are not a major source of carbon dioxide then it does not follow that they are largely responsible for the damage caused by global warming. Therefore A) is a valid assumption.

B) and C) are both stated in the question, whilst D) is irrelevant to the conclusion. E), meanwhile, is stated, as the question states that *we must now seek to curb air traffic in order to save the world's remaining natural environments*.

Question 11: B

A) and C) can be inferred, as the question states that these things would happen. Meanwhile, D) and E) actually serve to reinforce the argument's conclusion that the research into a new cure will not be successful. Therefore, they are not flaws in the argument's reasoning.

The point raised by B) does weaken the argument, and is a valid flaw in the argument's reasoning.

Question 12: E

A), C) and D) are all irrelevant to the argument's main conclusion, namely that Egypt was a powerful nation and must therefore have had a very strong military.

B) is a conclusion from the argument, but goes on to support E). If a nation required a very strong military to be a powerful nation, then it follows that if Egypt was a powerful nation it must have had a very strong military. Therefore, B) is an intermediate conclusion within the argument. E) is the *main* conclusion of the argument.

Question 13: D

At no point does the argument state or imply that we should not be concerned about damage to the polar ice caps, or that reducing energy consumption will not reduce CO2 emissions. Therefore, B) and E) are incorrect.

C) could be described as an assumption made in the argument, and is therefore not a conclusion.

A) goes beyond what the argument says. The argument does not say there are no environmental benefits to reducing energy consumption; it merely says it will not help the Polar Ice Caps. Therefore A) is incorrect and C) is a valid conclusion from the argument.

Question 14: C

A), B) and D) are all in direct contradiction to statements made in the passage, so cannot be conclusions. E), meanwhile, does not contradict the argument, but at no point does the argument say that the dangerous isomer was not effective at relieving nausea, so E) is not a conclusion.

However, the fact that the company followed the required level of testing and still did not detect the dangerous isomer does suggest that the required level of testing was not sufficient to identify isomers, so C) is correct.

Question 15: E

Ashley has to be sat in the front left seat so there are only two seats left in the front row. Bella and Caitlin have to be sat in different rows, so one of them must be sat in the front row and one in the back row. Now there is only one seat left in the front row, so there is not room for Danielle and her teaching assistant to both sit there. Therefore Danielle and the teaching assistant must take the two remaining seats in the back row. Therefore Emily must sit on the front row as there are no seats remaining in the back row. Emily cannot sit in the middle seat due to her mobility issues, so she must sit in the front right seat.

Question 16: A

At no point is it stated or implied that car companies should prioritise profits over the environment, so C) is incorrect. Neither is it stated that the public do not care about helping the environment, so E) is incorrect.

B) is a reason given in the argument, whilst D) is impossible if we accept the argument's reasons as true, so neither of these are conclusions.

Question 17: B

E) is contradictory to the main conclusion of the argument.

A), C) and D) are all reasons which go on to support the main conclusion of the argument, which is given in B). If we accept A), C) and D) as true, then it follows readily that the statement given in B) is true. Therefore, B) is the main conclusion.

Question 18: E

We can work out the code for each number and see which one equals 3.

The code for A is (3x4) = 12, divided by 6 = 2, minus 1 = 1

The code for B is (9x8) = 72, divided by 6 = 12, minus 4 = 8

The code for C is (5x4) = 20, divided by 2 = 10, minus 3 = 7

The code for D is (7x8) = 56, divided by 4 = 14, minus 8 = 6

The code for E is (6x8) = 48, divided by 4 = 12, minus 9 = 3

Therefore the pin number with the code 3 is E, 6839.

Question 19: C

The manager's conclusion (that the centre should hire Candidate 1 in order to maximise profits) relies on the assumption that performance experience, rather than welfare experience, will maximise profits. A valid flaw will mean that this assumption is not valid.

A) supports this assumption and so is not a flaw. B) is irrelevant as this assumption does not rest on the performance experience being with dolphins specifically. D) is irrelevant as it concerns a charity's outlook and is thus not relevant to a profit-making business. If E) were indeed a correct prediction then it could still be that profit would rise by *more* with Candidate 1, so the manager may still be correct.

C) is a flaw as it expresses a way in which profit may be higher if the business prioritises welfare standards over performance standards, as a boycott of the business could potentially greatly reduce profits.

Question 20: E

We can calculate all the rental yields as follows:

House A: (700x12)/168000 = 0.05

House B: (40x125x4)/200000 = 20000/200000 = 0.10

House C: (600*12)/144000 = 7200/144000 = 0.05

House D: (2000*12)/240000 = 24000/240000 = 0.10

House E: (200*52)/100000 = 10400/100000. We can see by observation that this is > 0.1 as 10000/100000 would equal 0.1, therefore there is no need to work this out to be able to say that this is the house with the highest yield.

Question 21: B

B) is an underlying assumption in the Transport Minister's argument. If rural areas have plenty of passengers, her assertion that rail companies will not run many services to these areas does not follow from her reasoning. Therefore, if B) is true, it strengthens the transport minister's argument.

Meanwhile, D) would actually weaken the transport minister's argument, suggesting that privatisation would not lead to less service for rural areas.

C) is irrelevant as the transport minister is arguing about how rural communities will be cut off by a privatised system. She is not referring to the quality or price of rail services under a publically subsidised system.

A) and E) are completely irrelevant points, which have no effect at all on the strength of the Transport Minister's argument.

Question 22: C

If it will cost Niall £2 more to pay per session than to buy membership, the combination of classes and gym sessions he is going to attend must cost £32. The only one of these combinations which costs £32 is C (5 x gym sessions at £4, 6 x classes at £2). Hence the answer is C.

Question 23: D

If the median is 6, the 3rd number when the numbers are written in order is 6. If the mode is 4, there must be at least two 4s (and can only be two 4s, because there are only 2 numbers less than 6 due to what we know about the median). Therefore, the smallest three numbers in the set are 4, 4, 6. For the mean to be 8, the numbers must add up to 5 times 8 = 40. Therefore the largest two numbers must add up to 40-(4+4+6)=26.

Question 24: A

B) and E) are irrelevant points which do not affect the strength of Lucy's argument.

C) and D) would both serve to strengthen Lucy's argument. C) suggests that running costs will be low, whilst D) suggests that visitor centres are profitable. Both of these, if true, serve to suggest that opening up visitor centres will be profitable for the park, therefore supporting Lucy's argument.

A), however, would weaken Lucy's argument by suggesting that visitor centres will not be profitable.

Question 25: E

There are 16 squares of dimension 1. There are 9 squares of dimension 2 (one in each corner, one halfway across each side and one right in the middle). There are 4 squares of dimension 3 (one in each corner). There is 1 square of dimension 4. Therefore, the total number of squares is $16 + 9 + 4 + 1 = 30$.

Question 26: D

If the announcement is accurate to the nearest 10 minutes, this means that the soonest the train will arrive in London is 115 minutes after the announcement, which is 17:25. The final destination is 10 minutes from King's Cross, so the earliest time I might arrive there is 17:35.

Question 27: C

When the sister's son is home, she has to buy a carton of washing powder 1.2 times as often, so she must be doing 1.2 times as many loads of washing. If we let x be the number of people living at home when the son is home, the number of loads of washing when he is home is 2+x, whereas the number when is not at home is 2+x-1=1+x. Therefore 2+x must equal 1.2(1+x). Rearranging this we get 0.8=0.2x, so x is 0.8 divided by 0.2, which is 4. So 4 people are living in the house when the son is home.

Question 28: D

The total time each train can run is 18 hours a day. Each journey takes the train 30 minutes (24+4+2). So each train can make 36 journeys a day. Therefore the total journeys made by the shuttle service per day will be 2x36 (because there are 2 trains) so the answer is 72.

Question 29: D

The lowest common multiple of 6, 4 and 2.5 is 60. Hence trains from all 3 lines will arrive at the same time every 60 minutes. If the last time they did was 4 minutes ago, it will hence be 60-4=56 minutes until they do so again. Therefore the answer is D.

Question 30: D

If Sam buys the invitations, she will spend £90 (90 x £1 each).

If Sam makes the invitations, she will need enough supplies for 94 invitations, which will be:

- 4 packs of red paper at £2 each = £8
- 7 rolls of ribbon at £3 each = £21
- 4 packs of gold stickers at £1 each = £4
- 1 stamper = £8
- 2 ink pads at £4 each = £8
- 5 packs of cream card at £2 each = £10

Adding these up, we get that the total spent on making the invitations herself is £59. Therefore she saves £90-£59=£31 by making them rather than buying them. Therefore the answer is D.

Question 31: B

If there are at least as many boys as girls in the class of 36, then there are at least 18 boys and at least 9 boys have brown eyes. If two thirds of the class have brown hair and at least as many boys as girls have brown hair, at least two thirds of the boys in the class have brown hair, so at least 12 boys have brown hair. There are only 18 boys in the class, so of the 9 boys who have brown eyes and 12 who have brown hair, at least 3 of these must be the same boys. So at least 3 boys in the class have both brown hair and brown eyes.

Question 32: C

The total amount of dilute squash needed is (300ml x 8) + (400ml x 3) = 3600ml. Mandy has 600ml of concentrated squash so she needs 3000ml of water to make up the right amount. There should be 3000ml:600ml of water:concentrated squash so the ratio needed is 5:1

END OF SECTION

Section 2

Question 1: B
Natural selection favours those who are best suited for survival – this can mean faster and stronger organisms, but not always. For example, snails are pervasive, despite being weak and slow. Variation can arise due to both genetic and environmental components.

Question 2: H
Chloride is oxidised during this process to form Cl_2. Although the first part of 2) is correct, H_2O is required to dissolve the NaCl (not H_2 which is a product of the reaction). NaOH is a strong base.

Question 3: D
The enzyme amylase catalyses the breakdown of starch into sugars in the mouth (1) and the small intestine (5).

Question 4: E
Whilst there is some enzymatic digestion in 1 and 3, the vast majority occurs in the small intestine (5). The liver facilitates digestion via the production of bile, and the large intestine is primarily responsible for the absorption of water.

Question 5: B
This is an example of an addition reaction, the fluorine and hydrogen atoms are added at the unsaturated bond. If you're unsure about this type of question draw it out and the answer will be obvious.

Question 6: D
The energy in a nuclear bomb comes from $E = mc^2$. When two nuclei fuse, the combined mass is slightly smaller than the two individual nuclei, and the mass lost is converted to energy according to Einstein's equation. Fusion releases much more energy than fission, as in the sun, and humans cannot harness this energy yet. Uncontrolled fission causes the explosion in an atom bomb and is created by a neutron-induced chain reaction. In power plants these neutrons are tightly controlled, so as not to overload the reactors and cause an explosion.

Question 7: A
The hydrogen halide binds to the alkene's unsaturated double bond. This results in a fully saturated product that consists purely of covalent bonds.

Question 8: B

$$\left(\frac{T}{4\pi}\right)^2 = \frac{l(M + 3m)}{3g(M + 2m)}$$

$$\frac{T^2}{16\pi^2} \times \frac{3g}{l} = \frac{M + 3m}{M + 2m}$$

$$3gT^2(M + 2m) = 16l\pi^2(M + 3m)$$

$$3gT^2M + 6gT^2m = 16l\pi^2M + 48l\pi^2m$$

$$6gT^2m - 48l\pi^2m = 16l\pi^2M - 3gT^2M$$

$$m(6gT^2 - 48l\pi^2) = 16l\pi^2M - 3gT^2M$$

$$m = \frac{16l\pi^2M - 3gT^2M}{6gT^2 - 48l\pi^2}$$

Question 9: A
The polymerisation reaction opens the double bond between the two C atoms to allow the formation of a long chain of monomers.

Question 10: A

Replotting the genetic diagram with genotype information produces the diagram:

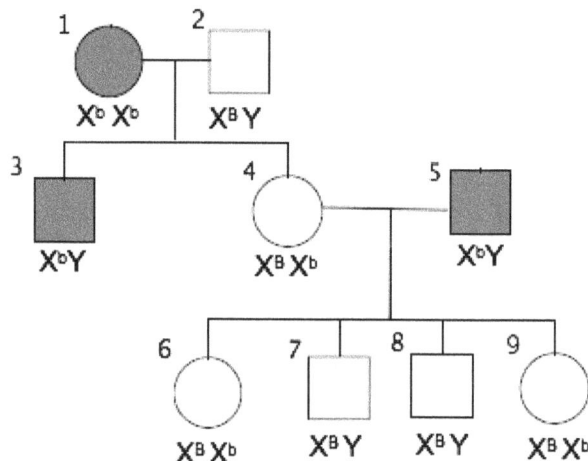

If squares were female, all of 5's circular male offspring would be affected. Circles must be females, so 1 must be homozygous recessive.

Question 11: D

The genotype of a heterozygote female is be $X^B X^b$, and the genotype of 8 is $X^B Y$. Plotting the information in a Punnett square:

		Female Heterozygote	
		X^B	X^b
Individual 8 (Unaffected Male)	X^B	$X^B X^B$	$X^B X^b$
	Y	$X^B Y$	$X^b Y$

The progeny produced are 25% $X^B X^B$ (homozygous normal female), 25% $X^B X^b$ (heterozygous carrier female), 25% $X^B Y$ (normal male) and 25% $X^b Y$ (affected male). So the chance of producing a colour blind boy is 25%.

Question 12: B

The mean is the sum of all the numbers in the set divided by the number of members in the set. The sum of all the numbers in the original set must be: 11 numbers x mean of 6 = 66. The sum of all the numbers once two are removed must then be: 9 numbers x mean of 5 = 45. Thus any two numbers which sum to 66 – 45 = 21 could have been removed from the set.

Question 13: F

All of the above are true. Every mole of gas occupies the same volume. The left side therefore occupies 4 volumes, and the right side occupies 2 volumes. Increasing pressure will favour the lower volume side, and the equilibrium will shift right to produce ammonia and decrease the overall volume that the products and reactants occupy. If more N_2 gas is added, equilibrium will shift to react away this gas and lower the concentration again, with the result that more ammonia will be formed.

Question 14: E
From the rules of angles made by intersections with parallel lines, all of the angles marked with the same letter are equal. There is no way to find if $d = 90°$, only that $b + d = c = 180° - a = 135°$, so b is unknown.

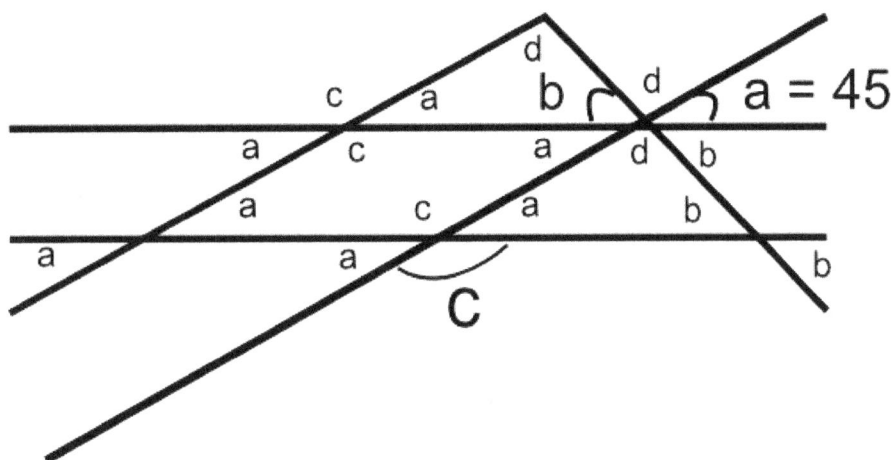

Question 15: E
Sodium is element 11 on the periodic table, a group 1 element, so has electron configuration: 2, 8, 1. It forms a metallic bond with other sodium atoms. Chlorine is element 17 in group 7, so has 17 electrons and 7 valence electrons, giving configuration: 2, 8, 7. Chlorine forms the covalent gas Cl_2, sharing one electron for a full valence shell.

Salt (NaCl) is an ionic compound, where sodium gives its single valence electron to chlorine so both atoms have full outer electron shells (8 electrons, so 2, 8:2, 8, 8).

Question 16: B
Let $y = 3.4 \times 10^{10}$; this is not necessary, but helpful, as the question can then be expressed as:
$$\frac{10y + y}{200y} = \frac{11y}{200y} = \frac{11}{200} = \frac{5.5}{100}$$
$$= 5.5 \times 10^{-2}$$

Question 17: B
As the known parent has both recessive genotypes, it can only have the gametes, y and t. The next generation has a phenotypic ratio of 1:1:1:1. As both recessive and dominant traits are present in the progeny, the unknown parent's genotype must contain both the recessive and dominant alleles. Hence the unknown parent's genotype must be YyTt as this would produce the gamete combinations of YT, Yt, yT and yt, which when combined with the known yt gametes would result in YyTt, Yytt, yyTt and yytt in equal ratios.

Question 18: D
The possible genotypes are: YYTT (yellow, tall), YyTT (yellow, tall), yyTT (green, tall), YYTt (yellow, tall), YYtt (yellow, short), YyTt (yellow, tall) Yytt (yellow, short), yyTt (green, tall), yytt (green, short). Thus, 9 different genotypes and 4 different phenotypes are possible.

Question 19: B
During electrolysis a current is used to draw charged ions to electrodes. The anode is positively charged and draws anions like sulphate, and the cathode is negatively charged and attracts positively charged cations like copper. For electrolysis to work well, the electrodes need to keep their positive or negative charge. If an alternating AC-current was used, the anode and cathode would repeatedly switch places, and the ions would make no net movement toward either electrode.

Question 20: C

Transform all numbers into fractions then follow the order of operations to simplify. Move the surds next to each other and evaluate systematically:

$$= \left(\left(\frac{6}{8} x \frac{7}{3}\right) \div \left(\frac{7}{5} x \frac{2}{6}\right)\right) x \frac{4}{10} x \frac{15}{100} x \frac{5}{100} x \frac{5}{25} x \pi x \left(\sqrt{e^2}\right) x e\pi^{-1}$$

$$= \left(\frac{42}{24} \div \frac{14}{30}\right) x \frac{4 \, x \, 3 \, x \, 25}{10 \, x \, 20 \, x \, 100 \, x \, 25} x \pi x \pi^{-1} x e^{-1} x e$$

$$= \left(\frac{21}{12} \div \frac{7}{15}\right) x \frac{12}{200 \, x \, 100} x \frac{\pi}{\pi} x \frac{e}{e}$$

$$= \left(\frac{21}{12} x \frac{15}{7}\right) x \frac{3}{50 \, x \, 100}$$

$$= \frac{45}{12} x \frac{3}{5000}$$

$$= \frac{9}{4} x \frac{1}{1000}$$

$$= \frac{9}{4000}$$

Question 21: B

R of series circuit= R + R = 2R

$$\text{R parallel} = \frac{1}{\frac{1}{R}+\frac{1}{R}} = \frac{1}{\frac{2}{R}} = \frac{R}{2}$$

Thus, the parallel circuit has a smaller resistance than the series circuit.
Since $I = \frac{V}{R}$, the parallel circuit will have a greater current than the series.

Question 22: D

Firstly, convert 36km/h to m/s to conserve units:
$$\frac{36,000 \, m}{3600 \, seconds} = \frac{360 \, m}{36s} = 10\frac{m}{s}$$

Before the driver can react the car travels at 36 km/hour for 0.5 seconds. Thus, it covers a distance of 0.5 x 10 = 5 metres.
There are 100 m left to the deer and the car must slow from 10 m/s to 0 m/s.
Using: $v^2 = u^2 + 2as$ gives: $0 = 10^2 + 2 \, x \, a \, x \, 100$
Thus, $-200a = 100$
Thus, $-200a = 100$
Thus, $a = -0.5 \, ms^{-2}$
Finally, using $F = ma$: $2000 \, x \, 0.5 = 1,000 \, N$

Question 23: D

Isotopes of an element all contain the same number of protons but a different number of neutrons. As atomic number refers solely to the number of protons it will not change. However as mass number is the sum of atomic number and neutron number – it would be expected to change. If an isotope contains one extra proton, then assuming that the charge of that isotope is 0, then it must also contain one extra electron. Chemical properties are the same for all isotopes. Therefore, the correct answer is D.

Question 24: C

Although the magnitude of acceleration decreases after 5 seconds he is still increasing his velocity. In this case, the velocity is given by the area under the curve. Summing the velocity gained over each second gives the final velocity, with squares here corresponding to 1 m/s² x 1 s = 1 m/s. He only ever loses velocity between 0-0.5 s and 9.5-10 s.

Question 25: C

The radius and tangent to a circle always form a right angle, so using Pythagoras:

$3^2 + 4^2 = X^2$
$X = 5$ m

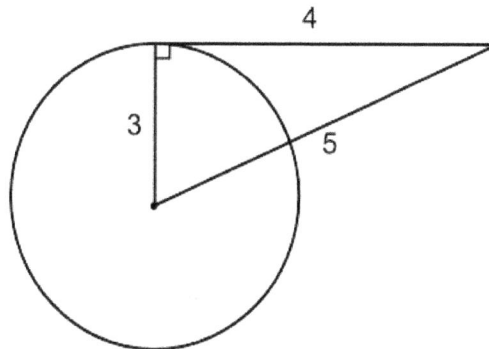

Question 26: E

Statements A, B and C are correct. Although energy is usually wasted when transformed, e.g. in power plants and engines, there are times when energy can be transformed without any losses to extraneous energy forms, e.g. a ball free-falling through a vacuum loses potential energy and gains kinetic energy without losses to other energy forms. Energy can be dispersed through vacuums e.g. solar heat energy through space.

Question 27: A

A beam of light is refracted toward the normal to the glass-air interface when it enters the glass, but refracted away by the same amount when it exists, for overall no net change. The angle of reflection of a beam is equal to (and thus dependent on) the angle of incidence. Beams of light entering a denser medium are refracted toward the normal to the interface, so light entering a pool of water would descend more steeply. Excited electrons in any atom can emit a massless photon to reduce their energy.

END OF SECTION

Section 3

'Doctors will eventually become obsolete as a result of advancing medical technologies.'

Explain what this statement means. Argue to the contrary. To what extent do you agree with the statement?

Technological advances in medicine are becoming increasingly important for modern diagnostics. Examples include X-ray technology and genetics, which both play an increasingly important role in medical diagnostics. Different forms of X-Ray imaging play a vital role in all medical investigations, whilst genetics are becoming increasingly important in finding tailored cures for complex diseases such as HIV, bacterial antibiotic resistance or even for cancer. The central idea underlying the statement is that knowledge and the ability to detect information on different patient parameters is all that is needed to cure him or her.

There is no doubt that increasing technological abilities play a central role in the treatment and diagnosis of disease. And in a sense, it is correct that the ability to accumulate a wide range of data will aid in the diagnosis of disease and therefore contributes to the treatment. But curing a disease goes beyond the mere diagnosis. A diagnosis will only allow the medical professional to decide on the path to take for treatment of the individual disease, but it will not necessarily facilitate a cure. Using HIV as an example, the ability to genetically detect implantation of the retrovirus in the cells DNA aids in making a diagnosis and the existence of anti-retroviral medication will allow for the suppression of the disease and allow the patient to lead an almost normal life, but even with all this knowledge and all these capabilities, owed to technological progress, a cure is not possible. But even in diseases that can theoretically be cured, the mere ability to cure it is worth little without the treating medical professional making the right decisions concerning investigations and treatments. Ultimately, the component of human error will never be outweighed by any technological ability and vice versa, the complexity of the human mind will never be replaced by machines.

The statement has some merit as technology is a central component of modern diagnostics and therefore is an important tool in pointing the treating medical professional into the right direction. It will however never replace experience and intuition from the side of the treating doctor as there will always be some degree of biological variance between patients that makes sole reliance on technological data difficult and potentially inaccurate. In essence, whilst technological means of diagnosis, and through this technological advance, play an important role in modern medicine and the cure of patients, it is unlikely for technological achievements to ever.

"Science is a procedure for testing and rejecting hypotheses, not a compendium of certain knowledge."

Stephen Jay Gould

What do you understand from the statement above? Explain why it might be argued that science does rely on a compendium of certain knowledge? To what extent is science defined by the challenging of preconceived hypotheses?

"A compendium of certain knowledge" refers to science as a self-contained, consistent body of information. Gould argues that rather than being static, science is the constant challenging of current ideas about the processes that underlie the universe. It is this idea of scientific controversy and continuous adaptation to new experimental findings that enables science to be driven forward, via the rejection of previous hypotheses and formulation of new ones.

However, many fundamental scientific ideas have been supported on so many occasions that they could be considered close to empirical truths. Since Darwin's formulation of the theory of natural selection, many natural observations have verified this theory, for example the observed selection of camouflaged peppered moths over white moths in the smog-filled Victorian Britain. Further understanding of inheritance, as being mediated through chromosomes has since led to the acceptance of natural selection within the scientific community.

Moreover, some scientific work is focused on determining the details of an accepted body of knowledge. Over twenty years of sequencing was undertaken by the Human Genomes Project to derive the full human genetic code. Rather than challenging any hypothesis, science in this case was working from the understanding that the human genome was the means of inheritance through its sequence of bases.

However, even though some scientific fundamentals are accepted, this does not mean they will eventually be challenged. The notion of classical mechanical physics was accepted as the ultimate explanation for all universal processes, for hundreds of years. It was only at the beginning of the 20th century where particles were shown to be able to display wave-like properties, that the concept of quantum physics was born. It is important to note that 'fundamental' scientific theories are *theories* – even scientific acceptance of natural selection has been updated to take into account new discoveries such as that of the inheritance of chemical alterations to DNA, epigenetics.

Newton summarises the work of science accurately: "If I have seen further it is by standing on the shoulders of giants". Scientific work often starts from the basis of a current body of knowledge, but ultimately it is the process of challenging this body that defines it – science is an ever-evolving, unconstrained field. However, as organisms limited to our five senses, perhaps science could be considered a compendium of knowledge, limited by our sense-based perception of the universe.

'Animal euthanasia should be made illegal'

Explain what this statement means. Argue to the contrary that animal euthanasia should remain legal. To what extent do you agree with the statement?

The statement argues that animal euthanasia, the act of humanely ending an animal's life or withholding life saving treatment, should be illegalised, usually on the grounds that it is cruel, unethical or inhumane. This essay will argue to the contrary that there are many instances in which animal euthanasia may be the best available option.

Firstly, there are many cases in which an animal may have a terminal illness such as cancer or rabies that would no longer respond to treatment. In these cases, it may be more humane to end the animals life in as swift and pain free a way as possible than to let it suffer helplessly for longer. Similarly, the animal may have a non-terminal illness, but one that may significantly affect its quality of life, or perhaps the owner could not afford the treatment. An animal's health and quality of life may significantly deteriorate in old age, and again, in these cases, euthanasia may be seen as the most humane option.

In some cases, the animal may suffer from behavioural problems that may mean that they are no longer suitable as a pet. While these problems may usually be corrected with the right care, in many instances, they fail to improve. A change in owner circumstances may mean that animals may have lack of a suitable home or caretaker. In both these cases, some people may believe that euthanasia is the kindest way to deal with them.

A large proportion of medical research is based on animal models. Euthanasia may be seen as the most humane way of killing animals in order to provide specimens for dissection, or to end animal suffering after experiments, with the balance being that the knowledge gained may result in better treatments overall for humans or animals.

In some instances such as with the foot and mouth outbreak in cows or tuberculosis in badgers, culling by euthanasia is crucial in spreading the spread of disease. Furthermore, population control of particular species e.g. Deers by euthanasia is crucial in maintaining particular ecosystems.

While I do believe it is morally wrong to end an animal's life unnecessarily, I largely disagree with the statement, I believe there are many instances, such as those described above, in which it is in the best interests of animals to be euthanized, and in these cases, it should remain legal.

'The primary duty of a doctor is to prolong life as much as possible'

What does this statement mean? Argue to the contrary, that the primary duty of a doctor is not to prolong life. To what extent do you agree with this statement?

This statement interprets medical beneficence as treating a patient so as to maximise their lifespan, irrespective of quality of life or the patient interests. This essay will argue that while prolonging life is a crucial part of a doctor's duty, it is not always the best, or most appropriate target of treatment.

Firstly, this statement assumes that all patients want to live longer. While it is a inherent quality of nature to want to survive, many patients, particularly elderly patients may feel they have already lived a long and fulfilling life and may not want to (in their eyes) artificially prolong their life further. They may rather wish to die naturally in their home surrounded by friends and family than in a medical setting.

The statement does not take into account any religious beliefs a patient may hold. For example, choosing to prolong the life of an unconscious patient with a blood transfusion may not be in the patients best interest if they were a Jehovah's witness, a sect of Christianity in which all blood products are banned as this may both compromise their beliefs and lead to them being banished from their community.

The statement also fails to address the issue of quality of life, instead simply choosing to focus on quantity. Is it worth having an extra five years of life if you were to be in excruciating pain or in a permanent vegetative state for the rest of it? The use of QALYs (quality adjusted life years) helps address this aspect, and for many patient, one extra year of disease free health may be more valuable than five extra years suffering.

In underfunded and stretched NHS where resources are finite, resource allocation also has to be considered when thinking about the duties of a doctor. On balance, some may say it is more just to spend £10,000 on providing life saving vaccination for hundreds of children than it may be to extend a 90 year olds life by a year.

While I do believe that prolonging life is, and always has been, one of the core aims of medicine, I do not agree that it is the primary duty of a doctor. I believe quality of life is equally as, if not more, important and should be taken into account. Furthermore, patient autonomy is one of the core principles of medicine and the patient's wishes should always be taken into account; if a patient applied for a DNR form previous to deteriorating, it would not be appropriate of a doctor to try prolong life as much as possible.

END OF PAPER

MOCK PAPER H ANSWERS
Section 1

Question 1: A

In this question we are looking at what cannot be reliably concluded from the passage. B and E conclude the state of a substance is not dependent on its chemical properties. C and D discuss how combining two substances can produce a new substance with very different physical properties. The passage refers to how the chemistry of a compound does not necessarily affect the physical properties of that compound. Thus, the answer must be A, which claims the chemical composition of a compound influences its physical nature.

Question 2: C

In this sequence, each alternate letter goes forward starting with B or backwards starting with Y. They start by jumping 4 letters, then 3, then 2 and finally the letters we are trying to find will have jumped by just 1. Thus, the letter after K is L, and the letter before P is O, so the answer is C.

Question 3: E

In this question we are looking at what can be reliably concluded from the passage. The passage is referring to products being made from similar parts; it is the way in which these parts are arranged that actually determines the final product. Thus, B cannot be right. D is also not correct, as there is no mention of protoplasm being the building block for life. E is the correct answer therefore.

Question 4: D

With these questions it is easiest to start at the end of the question and work backwards. The day two days before Monday is Saturday. The day immediately after that is Sunday. The day that comes four days after Sunday is Thursday, and two days after that is Saturday. Thus, the answer is D.

Question 5: D

In this question we are looking at what could weaken the passage above. The passage is discussing synthetic and natural cellulose and how their functions depend on whether the cellulose is plastic or colloidal. However, it states that the properties of natural and synthetic cellulose are equally similar. Therefore, any statement claiming some of the properties between the two forms of cellulose are different would weaken the passage, thus the answer is D.

Question 6: E

In order to work out this question, we need to make some simultaneous equations to relate John and Michael's money. If the amount of money John has at the start is J, and the amount that Michael has is M, we get the following equations:

$J - 20 = 2(M + 20)$ and $J + 5 = 5(M - 5)$, which is simplified to:

$J = 2M + 60$ and $J = 5M - 30$.

Substituting in, to work out M gives:

$2M + 60 = 5M - 30$, thus $3M = 90$ and $M = 30$.

Substituting in $M = 30$ to one of the equations gives:

$J = 60 + 60 = 120$.

Thus, $J + M = 150$, so the answer is E.

Question 7: E

In this question we want a summary of the passage. This passage refers to the use of fire in civilisations to create light. Through the passage it talks about the evolution of the use of fire, finishing with a reference to gas lamps in the street. Thus a good conclusion will refer to how the use of fire has changed over time, but also how lighting one's home is a key factor of civilisation. The answer must therefore be E, which discusses the evolution of fire use and also its importance in civilisation.

Question 8: A

972/2 = 486, thus 486 patients did not have chicken.

972/3 = 324, thus 162 patients did not have the chicken or the mac and cheese.

972/12 = 81, thus 972 – 486 – 324 – 81 = 81, which is the number of patients that had the vegetarian option. Therefore the answer is A.

Question 9: C

In this question we are looking at what can be reliably concluded from the passage. The passage does not tell us exactly how phosphorous was discovered, but we know that it was not Wilhelm Homberg who discovered it, thus A, B and D cannot be correct. 1669 is not in the 18th century thus E is also false. The passage describes how the element phosphorous was discovered by accident, by a man of low social status. Therefore, C is the only correct answer.

Question 10: D

For this question refer to the times in minutes, rather than hours, so 3pm is 180 minutes. x is the number of minutes past noon that we are trying to find. Therefore x + 28 will give the same amount of minutes past noon as 180-3x.

$x + 28 = 180 – 3x$

$4x = 152$

$x = 38$, thus the answer is D.

Question 11: B

In this question we are trying to find a suitable conclusion to the passage. A and E are completely irrelevant to the passage. C is incorrect as wings only attach to the posterior two segments of the insect's body. While D is correct, the legs are not referenced as being the most important part of the insect's body. Thus the answer must be B, which states the wings are the most dominant part of the body.

Question 12: D

For John: 56/64 x 100 = 87.5% or 7/8

For Mary: 24/36 x 100 = 66.7% or 2/3

Therefore we need to work out 7/8 – 2/3

21/24 – 16/24 = 5/24. Multiply by 100 to get the actual percentage:

500/24 = 125/6, thus the answer is D.

Question 13: A

To calculate this one needs to find the lowest common multiple of both 73 and 104, and then add that value to 2007. The lowest common multiple of 73 and 104 is 7592, which when added to 2007 gives 9559AD.

Question 14: D

In this question we are trying to find a suitable summary of the passage. There is no mention how important an animal is to mankind determining whether cruelty is acceptable, thus C and E are wrong. The passage states that the nature of the cruelty and the type of organism involved is irrelevant and should be punished regardless, thus the answer cannot be A or B, and must be D.

Question 15: B

If the number of girls is 40 more than the number of boys, and the boys make up 40% of the total number of students, then the discrepancy of 40 between boys and girls must represent 20%. Therefore, 1%=2 students and therefore the total number of students is 200.

Question 16: D

With this question it is easiest to start by putting the purple car between the green and the blue car. Since the red car is behind the blue car and the yellow car is in front of the green car, we know that the order of the cars must be:

Yellow, green, purple, blue and then red at the back.

Thus the second car in line is the green car and the answer is D.

Question 17: C

Based on the information, the school bus will get her to school at 09:01. The public bus arrives at 08:21, which she will miss, and the next bus will arrive at 08:38, which will take 18 minutes to arrive, meaning she will at school at 08:56, so the public bus at 08:38 will get her to school first.

Question 18: B

In this question we want a summary of the passage. The passage talks mostly about the feeding habits of the puddle duck, thus a summary discussing the predation of puddle ducks is irrelevant, meaning A and D are not correct. E is wrong as puddle ducks mainly live in shallow waters, and this is not because of their eating habits so C is also wrong. Thus, B is the correct answer as the ducks feed on mainly vegetarian food sources, and although they can dive for food, this is not their main route of feeding.

Question 19: A

In this question we want a summary of the passage. The veil discussed is clearly involved in a connection between the good and evil of the earth and therefore of mankind. Thus for a good summarising sentence, we want this connection to be discussed. Therefore, the answer must be A, which states that the veil links the good and evil of the human race, as is discussed in the passage.

Question 20: E

There is a specific sequence linking these numbers. Multiplying the first and third numbers of each row gives a number that makes up the second and fourth numbers of the same row.

9 x 3 = 27, thus the missing number is 7 and the answer is E.

Question 21: C

In this question we are looking to find the flaw in the argument. Answers D and E are irrelevant to the question. While B is correct it does not explain why the metformin inhibitor would have not had any effect on metformin's inhibition of fat cell growth. The key problem here is we are not given any information about the metformin inhibitor mentioned, and thus are not able to judge how it would affect metformin's fat cell growth inhibition, thus the answer is C.

Question 22:

We do not know whether Alexandra and Katie are dancers, so **A** and **B** are wrong. We do not know whether any dancers are ugly, so **D** is wrong.

Question 23: A

In this question, we are looking for a statement, which would support the passage. The reason that bacteriology has improved so much over recent centuries is due to our ability to study bacteria. Thus, any statement claiming our ability to study such organisms will support the passage. Therefore the answer must be either A or C. Techniques have improved out understanding of bacteria better than using antibiotics has, thus the answer must be A.

Question 24: C

Joseph is a man and no man is a lion i.e. all men are NOT lions hence Joseph is not a lion.

The statement is '1 to many' connection i.e. it puts Joseph in the bigger group of men BUT does not state that all men are or are not Joseph hence can't tell.

Question 25: D

In this question we are asked choose a sentence that most weakens the above argument. The main problem with this passage is that it struggles to give a reason for why water is not classified as a food. This is because the passage states that food is any nutriment that enters the body through the intestinal canal. Thus, water should be classified as food, but the passage claims that water is not food and does not give a reason for this. The answer is therefore D.

Question 26: C

Son age now= S
Father age now= F
$F- 4 = 4(S-4) -> F = 4S -12$
$F+6/S+6 =5/2 -> 2F +12 = 5S+ 30$
$8S -12 = 5S +30$
$S=14$
$F=44$

Question 27: D

In this question we are asked to find a conclusion for the passage. Not necessarily all metals and all metal salts form salts thus A and E are not correct. Treating tallow with acids forms a soap containing a metallic base not a metallic acid so E is false. Soaps are not just used for commercial use, driers and pharmaceutical preparations, which rules out B, therefore D is the correct answer as the basic definition of a soap in the passage is a fatty acid combined with a base.

Question 28: C

Total of 12 = $73*12=876$
$E + A + O = (73.6*15) – 876 = 228$
$68 +A + (A+6) =228$
$2A = 154 -> A=77$

Question 29: B

$90 x 8 x 120 = 86,400$. This value is the man hours required to get a third of the job done, therefore 172,800 man hours are required to finish the job. If they have 80 days left and 12 hours per day then:
$172,800/80 = 2,160$ and $2,160/12 = 180$, thus the answer is B.

Question 30: D

In this question we are asked to find a conclusion for the passage. The passage discusses how digestive tracts vary between mammals and describes how they differ between specific animals. This is presumably a result of the animals experiencing different environments and having different diets. Thus D is the correct answer.

Question 31: B

Letters a, c, e, g… will be lower case and B, D, F, H… will be upper case. Therefore, Wednesday will be written as weDNesDay, so the answer is B.

Question 32: B

Distance = 2/3S
distance=1-2/3S=1/3S
21/15 hr=2/3 S/4 + 1/3s /5
$84=14/3S * 3$
S= 6km

END OF SECTION

Section 2

Question 1: A

HCO_3^- is an alkaline substance and a vital component of the physiological buffering system. If the pH of the blood drops below 7, the bicarbonate molecule will accept a H^+ whereas if the pH increase, it will release H^+, thus HCO_3^- is an alkali.

Question 2: B

The current in a series circuit is always the same at any point in the circuit according to Kirchoff's first law which states that *at any node or junction in a circuit the sum of the current flowing into that node is equal to the current leaving that same node*. Thus current is always conserved. Since a series circuit does not have any nodes or junctions, we can assume the current is constant throughout.

The potential difference is shared between all the components of the circuit ($V_{total} = V_1 + V_2 + V_3...$). This is because the total work done on the charge by the battery must equal the total work done by the charge on the components. Resistance in a series circuit is the sum of all the individual resistances ($R = R1 + R2 + R3...$). The resistance of two or more resistors is bigger than the resistance of just one of the resistors on its own because the battery has to push charge through all of them.

Question 3: C

Solve as simultaneous equations

Start by substituting $x = \frac{y}{3}$ into equation B.

This gives $y = \frac{18}{y} - 7$

Multiply every term by y to give:

$0 = y^2 + 7y - 18$

Factorise this quadratic to give:

$0 = (y+9)(y-2)$

Where the graphs meet, y is equal to 2 and 9. Then y=3x so the graphs meet when x = 6 and x = 27

Question 4: B

There are several steps to working out this problem. The first is to work out the area of the entire floor, minus the fish tank and the cut out corner. We can see that the length of the room is 8m and the width of the room is 4m (the sides of the cut out square are 2m). Thus the area of the entire room is **32m²**.

The cut out corner is a square with the dimension 2 x 2m. Thus the area of the cut out corner is **4m²**.

The fish tank is a circle, and thus its area can be worked out using πr^2. Π is taken to be 3 and thus 3 x 1² = **3m²**. Therefore the floor area, Bill needs to cover is 32 – (4 + 3) = **25m²**.

We then need to work out the area of one plank. The dimensions of this are in cm and so we need to convert to m. 1m is 100cm and so we can say that the length of the plank is 0.6m and the width is 0.1m. Thus the area is 0.6 x 0.1 = **0.06m²**.

To work out the number of planks, required, we need to divide the area of the floor space by the area of the plank. A quick way of doing this would be rounding the area of the room down to 24 and multiplying the area of the plank by 100 so it becomes 6.

24/6 = 4, then because we multiplied the area of the plank by 100, we then multiply the answer by 100 which gives us **400 planks.** The closest answer to our solution is 417, which is listed as B.

Question 5: E

Some students may think that the arteries carry oxygenated blood from the mother to the foetus and that the vein carries the deoxygenated blood from the foetus to the mother, but it is important to remember that arteries always carry blood to the heart (in this case the mother's) and veins always travel away from the heart. A prime example of this is the pulmonary system, as like the foetal-mother system, the pulmonary arteries carry deoxygenated blood to the lungs away from the heart and the pulmonary veins carry oxygenated blood back to the heart.

Question 6: B

Solve $y = x^2 - 3x + 4$ and $y - x = 1$ as (x,y).

Substitute the quadratic expression into the other non-quadratic. You'll get another equation.

$x + 1 = x^2 - 3x + 4$

Rearrange to get a quadratic equation and solve.

$x^2 - 4x + 3 = 0$

$(x - 1)(x - 3) = 0$

Therefore x = 1 or x = 3

Substitute your x values into the equation, $y - x = 1$ and solve to work out y values.

y = 2 or y = 4

Therefore the coordinates are (1, 2) and (3, 4)

Question 7: B

Equate the volume with the surface area in the proportion instructed by the question. $3(^4/_3\pi r^3) = 4\pi r^2$, simplifies to r = 1.

Question 8: C

ΔH is positive because the enthalpy of the products is higher than the enthalpy of the reactants. This also means that the reactants are less stable than the products and because it is ENDOthermic, energy is absorbed from the surroundings.

Question 9: H

The kidneys are involved in ultrafiltration as they filter all of the blood in the body of toxins/waste products from metabolic reactions. The waste is released as urine via the bladder. Some of the water is filtered out then reabsorbed by the kidney, especially when the body is dehydrated. Although glucose is reabsorbed by the kidney, it does not play a part in glucose regulation as that is mainly done by the pancreas by secretion of insulin and glucagon. These hormones are two of many found in the body, none of which are produced by the kidneys. There are some that are produced by the adrenal cortices that sit atop the kidneys, but these are a separate anatomical structure from the kidney.

Question 10: A

Haemophilia B is an X-linked recessive disorder which means you need two copies of the faulty genes in girls to present the phenotype associated with the disease and only one copy in males as they have XY chromosomes and are thus missing the extra X chromosome which may have carried the healthy, dominant gene. As Mike, the father of the baby girl, is not affected, we can assume that the mother carries one copy of the faulty gene herself. Thus, although the baby girl will not be affected by the condition, she may be a carrier of the gene and so, can pass it on to future generations.

Question 11: A

There are several methods to work this out, one of which is shown below.

Mass of FeS_2 in the ore = 480 x 0.75 = 360kg

1 mole of FeS_2 = 55 + 32 + 32 = 119g → this can be rounded to 120g for ease of calculation.

Number of moles of FeS_2 in the ore = $\frac{360 \times 10^3}{120}$ = 3 x 10^3 mol

Mass of Fe = (3 x 10^3) x 55 = 165kg.

167.7kg is closest to this value.

Question 12: B

potassium	most reactive	K
sodium		Na
calcium		Ca
magnesium		Mg
aluminium		Al
carbon		C
zinc		Zn
iron		Fe
tin		Sn
lead		Pb
hydrogen		H
copper		Cu
silver		Ag
gold		Au
platinum	least reactive	Pt

Here, it is important to remember the reactivity series.

This is important as it tells you which elements are able to displace other elements in redox reactions. In this example, Zinc is the only element above Iron in the series and thus, is the only element that would be able to displace Iron.

Question 13: A

As galaxies and celestial objects move away from Earth, the wavelength of the light they emit, gets longer as it travels towards us. Thus there is a noticeable shift towards the red end of the spectrum, when we measure those waves. Scientists are able to measure the real light coming from galaxies far away using telescopes that pick up and record this light. Using red shift we can tell which galaxies are further away and which ones are closer. There is another phenomena called blue shift, which is the opposite of red shift in that, we can tell which galaxies are moving closer to us as the wavelengths of those galaxies become shorter and therefore shift to the blue end of the spectrum.

Question 14: A

X-rays are able to pass through soft, less dense material, like skin, soft tissue and air to stain the x-ray film black. They can't pass through denser material like bone and thus the x-ray film stays white. X-rays are harmful with prolonged exposure as they ionise cells and cause DNA damage that can result in conditions like cancer. Radiologists or technicians working with x-rays wear lead aprons to protect them from excess radiation. Gamma rays are different to x-rays with shorter wavelengths that are able to pass through dense material and because of this, they are considered more dangerous than x-rays.

Question 15: A

$\frac{(16x+11)}{(4x+5)} = 4y^2 + 2$

$16x + 11 = (4y^2 + 2)(4x + 5)$

$16x + 11 = 4x(4y^2 + 2) + 5(4y^2 + 2)$

$16x - 4x(4y^2 + 2) = 5(4y^2 + 2) - 11$

$x(16 - 4(4y^2 + 2) = 20y^2 - 1$

$X = \frac{20y^2 - 1}{[16 - 4(4y^2 + 2)]}$

Question 16: A

In the diagram shown, the number at the top (73) denotes the mass number of an atom of Germanium. This is the number of protons and neutrons in the nucleus. The number at the bottom (32) is the proton number, i.e. the number of protons in the nucleus. Protons have a positive charge, neutrons have a neutral charge and electrons have a negative charge. As a stable element, Germanium must have a charge of 0 and thus the electrons and protons have to cancel out. Therefore, Germanium has 32 electrons.

Question 17: F

The first line defence of the body from invading pathogens is the skin. This is a tough keratinized layer, which is not easily broken down by bacteria. There is also flora on the skin (bacteria that live on the skin) that prevents any harmful bacteria from colonising. The next line of defence is the mucus lining the airways. It traps dirt and pathogens, to be either expelled from the body or swallowed into the gut. The next layer of defence mentioned in the answers, is hydrochloric acid found in the stomach. This has a pH of 2 and so effectively kills any pathogens that enter the body through the food. Other defences not listed include, tears (they contain lysozymes that break down the bacteria) and acidic substances by the sebaceous glands of the skin.

Some students may get confused by the antibodies. Although it is true that antibodies provide a line of defence, they are a secondary line of defence after the pathogen has got past the initial defences.

Question 18: D

The first step is to multiply out $(3p + 5)^2$

$(3p + 5)(3p + 5) = 24p + 49$

$9p^2 + 30p + 25 = 24p + 49$

$9p^2 + 6p - 24 = 0$

Then put the quadratic into brackets.

$(3p + 6)(3p - 4) = 0$

Therefore p must equal -6 or +4.

Question 19: G

The collision theory applies to all materials in any state that are reacting with each other. Increasing the temperature of a system increases the kinetic energy of the particles, making them move faster and this increases the force of collisions as well as the chance of two or more particles colliding. Increasing the smaller area of the substance reacting (making the particles smaller e.g. solids become fine powders or liquid become gases) increases the chances of more collisions happening. Another way to increase collisions is by increasing the pressure of a system as the molecules are in a more enclosed space and thus have less room to move without colliding with each other.

Question 20: E

Aluminium is not a good conductor of heat and thus heat is preserved. It is also shiny and thus is a poor emitter and absorber of heat. This means it won't let heat out, nor will it cause the person to overheat.

Question 21: C

Osmosis is the movement of water particles across a partially permeable membrane from an area of low concentration to an area of high concentration (of solute). It is not an active process as water can easily diffuse through bilipid layer membranes and thus does not require a specific passage.

Question 22: A

This is complete combustion as all of the methane is used to make water and carbon dioxide. It is an aerobic reaction as oxygen is present and needed to cause the combustion of the fuel. By increasing the carbon dioxide in the system you would either slow down or not affect the rate of combustion, but definitely would not speed it up. This also applies to removing oxygen from the system.

Question 23: A

Recall that R = V/I which is Ohm = Volt/Ampere which is expressed as $V.A^{-1}$.

Question 24: D

The equation for work done is: W (Nm) = F (N) x d (m)

Therefore, substituting the information available in the question, you can rearrange the equation and work out the answer:

40 = F x 0.2

40/0.2= F

200 = F

Question 25: B

Plants also give off carbon via respiration and death. Although some of the carbon is given off, trees and plants do store carbon in their cells and thus they are known as carbon stores.

Question 26: B

If a wave hits a boundary at an angle, it will refract because, the part of the wave that hit the boundary first slows down before the rest of it. This causes it to change direction and speed as demonstrated below:

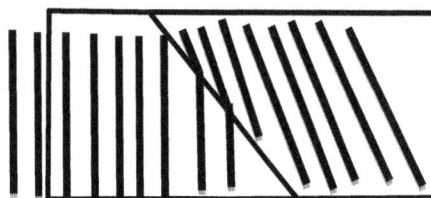

If a wave hits a boundary face on, it does not change direction, but slows down as demonstrated below:

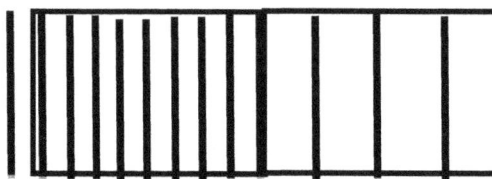

Waves slow down if they hit a boundary from low density to high density.

Question 27: A

Enzymes are always substrate specific as the active site is made up of a specific set of amino acids that determine which reaction the enzyme catalyses.

END OF SECTION

Section 3

1) **"Time and time again, throughout the history of medical practice, what was once considered as "scientific" eventually becomes regarded as "bad practice"."** – David Stewart

What does this statement mean? Give some examples of times when scientific practice has become bad practice and describe how this has had an impact on medicine.

This statement seems to suggest that as medicine and science progress, there is a constant change in the way healthcare professionals treat and manage various conditions. For example, until recently, the use of Sodium Valproate as a drug to treat epilepsy had been highly effective but it was found to cause congenital abnormalities in the growing foetus and thus it is now considered 'bad practice' to prescribe Sodium Valproate during pregnancy.

Change is crucial if we want to improve and advance the way we treat and practice in medicine. Science is constantly discovering new things and disproving previously accepted theories. With this information being easily accessible over the internet, it is key that we as healthcare providers ensure we don't lag behind and provide the newest, most effective treatments available for our patients. Not only does this increase patient satisfaction, it also increases patient safety as practices that have previously been safe in one patient population may not be safe in another.

A good example of this, along the same vein as Sodium Valproate, is Thalidomide. Used as a drug to treat conditions such as Leprosy and TB, it was found to be a highly effective antiemetic and was prescribed for women as a treatment for morning sickness. Unfortunately, the drug was not tested thoroughly enough to determine its effects on the growing foetus and many babies were born with congenital abnormalities, namely missing limbs. The outcome of this disaster was a worldwide effort to bring about stricter drug licensing and testing regulations. It is now bad practice to prescribe drugs without knowing the full extent of its adverse effects. This has brought about a practice in which everyone has benefited, both patients and healthcare providers.

Another example of scientific processes becoming bad practice is the Andrew Wakefield MMR scandal. Wakefield conducted a study on the correlation between autism and the MMR vaccine in young children. His study seemed to prove that there was a strong correlation which led to many parents refusing to vaccinate their children. This caused an epidemic of MMR across the country. After researchers reviewed his study and found that his study was in fact inaccurate and the results were forged, MMR vaccine uptake rates started to increase and the incidence of MMR decreased drastically. This has changed both scientific and medical practice as any research that is available is peer reviewed and carried out to the highest standard to avoid such instances like this.

In conclusion, change is needed, and it only serves to improve the service and the way we practice medicine today. Without 'bad practice' you do not have 'good practice' and as science and the world advances, it is important to remember that patient safety is always the most important part of medicine.

2) **"Formerly, when religion was strong and science weak, men mistook magic for medicine; now, when science is strong and religion weak, men mistake medicine for magic." – Thomas Szasz**

What does this statement mean? Do you think it is correct in assuming that all men mistake medicine for magic?

This statement suggests that the understanding of how medicine works is based upon the strength of science and what it can provide for the medical community. It portrays the idea that in the past, when religion was seen as the 'law,' people saw magic as miraculous cures for diseases and illnesses they didn't understand. Now that science has advanced and is seen in parallel with religion, or even as a competitor, people see medicine as something that provides the cures or the treatments to make them better. Because they don't fully understand the processes that occur in the body when medicine or treatment is prescribed, they perceive it as 'magic.'

In the past, we did not have access to knowledge about DNA or bacteria. Antibiotics were unheard of and any medical treatment given in the past was mainly trial and error. This resulted in patient deaths and a general sense of hopelessness – if a person fell ill, they were more likely to die. When someone happened to cure a person by chance, or they got better, it was seen as magic, forces of unknown nature and power being used to treat the individual. As science progressed and the world came to know more about the world around us and how we could utilise it to better ourselves, medicine also advanced. The medical world is still evolving, helped along by science as theories are disproved and new hypotheses are created. This leads to a level of awe as medicine starts to treat the untreatable or cure the incurable.

This is both beneficial and a hindrance to medicine. One benefit of medicine as magic is it demands a certain level of respect. Patients are willing to listen to healthcare providers and the advice we give as they know that medicine will help them. On the other hand, patients sometimes believe that they are entitled to this treatment and when it doesn't work, or cannot be prescribed, they get angry. One example of this is antibiotics. Many patients don't understand that antibiotics do not treat viral infections and demand the drugs in order to cure a cold or a sore throat. Sometimes despite an explanation of why antibiotics can't be prescribed, the patient still demands the antibiotic and the doctor has no other choice but to give in. This unnecessary overuse of antibiotics leads to antibiotic resistance which causes a grievance to the rest of the population.

In conclusion, we must be careful to educate our patients about aspects of medicine they may not understand. We must ensure that they do not hold medicine on too high a pedestal as that leads to decreased satisfaction and a sense of being let down. It is important that patients understand that medicine cannot cure everything, that medicine is the result of years of research and discovery, and that it takes time to evolve.

3) *"Approximately 26.9% of the adult population in the UK is obese. Shouldn't we be offering bariatric surgery to every obese person that walks through the doors?"*

Explain what this statement means. Argue to the contrary. To what extent do you agree with the statement?

Obesity is a major cause of heart disease, stroke, osteoarthritis, diabetes and much more. These conditions can lead to death, which is why it is important for people to lose weight.

Although losing weight is important, surgery is invasive and carries its own risks, like infection and bleeding. It is better to try to lose weight through diet and exercise first before trying invasive treatments. Diet and exercise are usually sufficient enough to cause a reduction in weight, and there are many ways a clinician can encourage his/her patients. Suggesting that the patient take it step by step (e.g. walking for ten minutes one day then walking fifteen minutes the next). This can make the task seem less daunting and the patient will be more likely to try and start losing weight this way. It also means that they ease themselves into it, and let their body adjust to the change. Supplementary interventions can include counselling which will probe into the patient's reasons for weight loss and encourage them.

If exercise and diet change are not working then certain drugs can be brought into play, which along with the diet and exercise help the patient reduce their BMI. However, medications have their own side effects, which can be unpleasant for the patient. These can deter the patient from taking them in which case, the clinician may need to look for alternatives or prescribe medication that counteracts the side effects.

Surgery is the last resort intervention as it is invasive and has the worst complications. Bariatric surgery is useful in that it is an easy way to help patients lose weight quickly along with exercise and diet changes. It can also make the patient more incentivised to carry out the weight loss plan as they may feel that the journey is shorter and will happen quicker.

This is counter-balanced by the fact that patients often have to lose weight before they go into surgery to minimise the risk of complications that occur afterwards. This means that although, surgery is easier and quicker than just exercise, a certain amount of weight loss will be required as a pre-requisite to the surgery and so patients will find that they have to exercise anyway.

In conclusion, surgery should not be offered to everyone who walks through the doors as not only is it expensive, it also has a lot of requirements and complications that can be very harmful to some. It is always better to encourage the patient to try non-invasive methods first then, if absolutely necessary use the invasive treatments.

4) *'Placebos may solve the problem of patients demanding medication they do not need.'*

Explain what this statement means. Argue the contrary. To what extent do you agree with the statement?

Placebos are used in research as a control against drugs that are being studied. They can either be sugar pills or a drug that has already been licensed and is known to treat the disease being studied by the researchers.

Patients often come into a GP consultation or to the hospital and expect a drug to be given to them, even when they don't need it. Millions of pounds are spent giving antibiotics to patients who have a viral infection and this costs the NHS greatly. The reason these are given is because although clinicians try to explain why antibiotics are not needed for viral infection, patients refuse to listen and demand the drugs anyway. In this case a placebo would reduce the overall harm caused by giving antibiotics out wrongly. Simple sugar pills would not harm the patient and would reduce the amount of abuse clinicians get for refusing to prescribe medication.

Placebos have also been shown to have a psychological effect on patients in that, patients feel better after having taken the placebo even if it was just a sugar pill. This could have a significant effect on care as placebos could help patients get better by themselves. Taking a pill makes the patient believe they are being treated and so in effect, they will themselves better. This would save the NHS a lot of money in the long run as less drugs and time would be used treating patients for whom the illness is easy to cure without medication.

The downside to placebo treatment is that the doctor-patient relationship may be harmed if the patient realises they are being given placebos. A certain level of trust is built up between the doctor and the patient, and regaining it is hard. Trust is paramount in the successful treatment of a patient. Another downside is that it is unethical to provide a placebo to a patient and make them believe they are actually being treated. It is dishonest and goes against the values of being a good doctor.

Overall, placebos should not be used as an alternative treatment as the pros do not justify the ethical dilemmas faced by a clinician. Trust is important in the relationship a doctor holds with a patient and that should take first priority. I think doctors should try and explain to their patients the best they can, that sometimes medication is not necessary to treat a certain disease/condition.

END OF PAPER

FINAL ADVICE

Arrive well rested, well fed and well hydrated

The BMAT is an intensive test, so make sure you're ready for it. Unlike the UKCAT, you'll have to sit this at a fixed time (normally at 9AM). Thus, ensure you get a good night's sleep before the exam (there is little point cramming) and don't miss breakfast. If you're taking water into the exam then make sure you've been to the toilet before so you don't have to leave during the exam. Make sure you're well rested and fed in order to be at your best!

Move on

If you're struggling, move on. Every question has equal weighting and there is no negative marking. In the time it takes to answer on hard question, you could gain three times the marks by answering the easier ones. Be smart to score points- especially in section two where some questions are far easier than others.

Make Notes on your Essay

Some universities may ask you questions on your BMAT essay at the interview. Sometimes you may have the interview as late as March which means that you **MUST** make short notes on the essay title and your main arguments after the essay. This is especially important if you're applying to UCL and Cambridge where the essay is discussed more frequently.

Afterword

Remember that the route to a high score is your approach and practice. Don't fall into the trap that *"you can't prepare for the BMAT"*– this could not be further from the truth. With knowledge of the test, some useful time-saving techniques and plenty of practice you can dramatically boost your score.

Work hard, never give up and do yourself justice.

Good Luck!

Acknowledgements

I would like to thank Rohan and the UniAdmissions Tutors for all their hard work and advice in compiling this book, and both my parents and Meg for their continued unwavering support.

Matthew

About Us

Infinity Books is the publishing division of *Infinity Education Ltd*. We currently publish over 85 titles across a range of subject areas – covering specialised admissions tests, examination techniques, personal statement guides, plus everything else you need to improve your chances of getting on to competitive courses such as medicine and law, as well as into universities such as Oxford and Cambridge.

Outside of publishing we also operate a highly successful tuition division, called UniAdmissions. This company was founded in 2013 by Dr Rohan Agarwal and Dr David Salt, both Cambridge Medical graduates with several years of tutoring experience. Since then, every year, hundreds of applicants and schools work with us on our programmes. Through the programmes we offer, we deliver expert tuition, exclusive course places, online courses, best-selling textbooks and much more.

With a team of over 1,000 Oxbridge tutors and a proven track record, UniAdmissions have quickly become the UK's number one admissions company.

Visit and engage with us at:

Website (Infinity Books): www.infinitybooks.co.uk

Website (UniAdmissions): www.uniadmissions.co.uk

Facebook: www.facebook.com/uniadmissionsuk

Twitter: @infinitybooks7